IMAGINATION
AND MEDICINE

IMAGINATION AND MEDICINE

The Future of Healing in an Age of Neuroscience

Edited by
Stephen Aizenstat and
Robert Bosnak

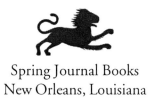

Spring Journal Books
New Orleans, Louisiana

Published by:
Spring Journal, Inc.
627 Ursulines Street #7
New Orleans, Louisiana 70116
Tel.: (504) 524-5117
Website: www.springjournalandbooks.com

Cover design:
Sherrie Lovler and Anthony Lawlor
Contact Sherrie Lovler at www.inkmonkey.com
Email sherrie@inkmonkey.com
Contact Anthony Lawlor at www.anthonylawlor.com
Email anthony@anthonylawlor.com

Cover photograph:
Serpent in Eden from the Portal of the Virgin,
Notre Dame Cathedral, Paris by Anthony Lawlor

Printed in Canada
Text printed on acid-free paper

ISBN 978-1-882670-62-8
Library of Congress Cataloging-in-Publication Data Pending

*To the Future of
the Ever Present Spirit
Asklepios*

Contents

HEALING SPACE

Preface

Imagine a campus overlooking the Pacific Ocean, the late-spring sun against a pale blue sky. About 250 people at a conference on *Imagination and Medicine* are milling about, awaiting a group of speakers of extraordinary variety and unique vantage points who will discuss a bedrock question: What are the forces that stimulate the body's capacity to heal itself? The self-healing response has ever been one of the great mysteries of medicine. Hippocrates tells us that it is the task of the doctor to assist the body in its innate process of regeneration.

In the previous century, Western medicine witnessed a series of heroic triumphs—along with failures—of disease-fighting technology. Methods of triggering self-healing moved into the background.

However, in this volume you will hear how advanced contemporary science finds overwhelming proof, in studies of the placebo effect and research in gene behavior, of imagination's much greater role in the healing process than one might have expected in the era of rational scientific medicine.

In addition to such contemporary findings as the dramatic effects of emotional trauma and stress upon the brain, scholars address indigenous healing in a variety of cultures, the significant role of dreaming at the beginnings of Western medicine, the ancient role of music in many systems of medicine, and the great importance of location and architecture in our places of healing.

The meeting of hearts and minds around the place of imagination in the practice of medicine was seeded by a decade of conversation between Robert Bosnak and me. Might it might be possible, we wondered, to create a place of healing that, in combination with conventional Western medicine, could serve to help the body heal itself? How might we employ the powers of creative imagination and the spirit of place, as had been invoked in the classical world when the healing god Asklepios was still afoot? We both had been strongly influenced by the central importance in classical medicine of dreaming and wished to reclaim such an emphasis for our age. Enhancing the power of conventional medicine by stimulating the body's self-healing tendencies would surely be more effective than administering conventional medicine as a stand-alone practice, we hypothesized.

We realized that it was time to expand the conversation between doctors fighting illness and those focused on the creative abilities of the body to heal itself. Hence, *Imagination and Medicine*—the conference and now the book.

We need to think together about what it takes to create healing environments that encourage the self-healing the body excels at, all the while fighting disease. We need to rekindle classical medicine, when imagination and technology walked hand in hand.

This book is a first step.

—STEPHEN AIZENSTAT

Coming to a Door

A Conversation with

M A R I O N   W O O D M A N

I think psychological factors are extremely important in healing because psyche and soma are virtually one. If psyche is ill, for example, if it is extremely depressed, if it is rejecting reality, whatever the reason for the depression, that will go into body, and body will pick it up into symptoms. That is certainly what I have observed with cancer. Where psyche is not at peace with body, where there is impending loss, impending illness in a family or the possibility of death is looming, that is an area where cancer can come in and be devastating.

The physical ailment can come in, but I suspect, from the many dreams I have worked with in my practice, that the psyche is ahead of the body. I remember one woman came to me one day; she had a drawing with her of what she had seen in a dream the night before. It was a Y shape, and there was a big bird's nest on top of the crux of the Y. Then there was a huge blackbird that pounced on top of that. The lady threw the drawing on the floor, and was so angry with this vision that had come in her dream that she yelled, "That's my mother sitting on my sexuality." There was also a horrible purple hand in this drawing. Part of me drew back from it. I told her if I had had that dream, I'd see a doctor on the way home. So she stopped at her doctor's office, whereupon her doctor told her that he didn't see anything, but since she was so upset, he would check her further. Sure enough she had cancer. The doctor was astonished that she was able to pick it up so quickly. The cancer was a long way from actually manifesting, but the dreams were manifesting from the beginning. Psychologically it was her mother sitting on her sexuality; the dreams were working to release her from that enslavement to the negative mother.

I think the image is the connector between psyche and soma. The feeling-tone in the body, where the belly resonates with the resonating heart and liver, all of this is producing chemistry that is picked up by the brain. Science is now working on this grand computer, the brain, transforming feeling into image. The image gives us an understanding of what's happening in the body and some insight into the anguish in the brain and the psyche. I see psyche and soma as one. The metaphorical symbol is the connector. It requires resonating space in which to unfold.

The tone of a consulting office has to be calm and cherishing. Patients come into an office having been battered around by the workplace, by the noise in the street, by the stink of the street; they have come to a place of healing when they enter the office. The subtle body knows if there has been anger in the office, knows what has been released in the session previously. Quiet, peaceful, colorful images can be unconsciously picked up through pictures on the walls. My feeling about an analytical session is that there has to be one moment of now, as Emily Dickinson says, "the perfect moment," when you are not cluttered by the past or the future; you simply are, present tense, verb to be. In that moment you can see yourself as you are. Not as your mother wanted you to be, not as your father wanted you to be, no one. The question is, "Who am I when all those crutches are removed?" A place where nobody has an agenda for me. It's simply, "Who am I?" That is the moment of "noon." I like to have the entire atmosphere contributing to that moment of silent knowing.

I think in the last twenty years there has been a huge advance in the acceptance of imagery as connector between body and soul. When I was in the hospital with cancer I was made fun of for not using the painkiller machine. Doctors and nurses asked whether I didn't know how to use the machine. When I told them I didn't need it, they wanted to know what was wrong with me. I tried to explain that I was connecting to imagery that could help me without all the drugs. They just shrugged their shoulders and thought I was crazy. Similarly with the whole healing process. However, as time went on, my doctor told me that he didn't know what I was doing with that "imagery stuff" but to keep on doing it. At that time imagery was iffy. No one that I met in the medical profession respected imagery. MRI machines have changed that. But imagery can change disease. I learned this while teaching school, through poetry. I learned it through kids who were impossible to handle, the so-called "terminal kids" (I hated that because they were really good kids with a terrible background). I used to have them memorize poems: fierce poems, like "The Tiger" by William Blake or by T. S. Eliot from "The Waste Land." They would memorize the poems and as they were reciting "Tiger! Tiger! burning bright / In the forests of the night" they would hold a ball and then fling it with such force, they ended up getting all that energy behind that ball into Tiger. Eventually, they were able to sit down and work with Julius Caesar! When they had a chance to do Mark Antony's speech, they all memorized that and they were ready to put their yardsticks in the air! That is where I learned the power of metaphor. And now in hospitals, certainly all over our country, all over our province anyway, they are working with metaphors as a healing tool.

I think anybody in analysis is working on dream incubation. If they are spending money to go to a session, if they don't have dreams, they are not getting the best of their session. They are not relating to their own unconscious. Most people in Jungian analysis set it up that they go to bed at a decent time, that they do not use an alarm clock that will rape the dream, and they try to get the dream written down during the night. Some dreamers use their voice-activated tape recorder and get two or three great dreams during the night. Because, you see, when you get into the deep REM sleep, it becomes very hard to get those dreams, but they are the big ones. Simple example: if you write dreams down, you say something like, "Yesterday I went to see my father." But if you spoke on the edge of wakefulness, it might come out something like, "I went to see my father . . . my father. I went to see my father." Then it means something totally different because you experience the feeling in the gut, the imagination, and the image of your father-totality. The body, the psyche—it all comes together in that image.

Yes, I am a Jungian analyst and I work with the body all the time. I have workshops where we are doing as much bodywork as we are doing dream interpretation. But certainly, as I said earlier with the story about the patient with the drawing of the Y, the moment I mentioned the Y and the big, black bird's nest, she was able to accept her immediate reality of the image. Certainly it made an immense difference in her healing process. For older people that I am working with now, and for me, dreams are a huge consolation. Because of the changes that are going on in their bodies and the fact that death is in the environment, we know that life can change in one instant, and so there is often anxiety, depression, or failure to relate. Then, in the dream, they may experience an image of coming to a door. They have to ask, "Do I open it or do I not open it?" Immense fear around that question! It may be left as a question mark in the dream. Sometimes I say, "I'll go through it with you"—and behold, there is a most marvelous road when we open the door. And sometimes there is nothing. And that's when we quietly shut the door until another time . . . .there will be a time. So yes, I would say it works both ways: In working with body, psyche can be healed; in working with psyche, body can be healed. They are together, beloved partners on the journey.

The Physician Inside

ROBERT   BOSNAK

Life is short and the art is long; the opportunity fleeting, experiment dangerous, and judgment difficult.

—Hippocrates

It was just after 9/11 and our world had changed, once again. My friend Stephen Aizenstat and I sat around drinking sake in a Japanese restaurant in Santa Barbara. My personal life had been turned upside down with my decision to move from the United States to Australia, and we talked about the future, what we still wanted to do in life: taking stock, you might say. To our surprise, we found that we were both fascinated by the Greek god Asklepios and his healing temples. Each of us had, independently, taken a group to Epidaurus, the god's primary sanctuary, to work with dreams—which is our trade.

What if, we mused, helped along by the spirit of rice, we started such a medical healing sanctuary, in drastically modified form but along the same principles, in Santa Barbara?

The Asklepian tradition pivots around the divine power of imagination that can transform a body out of illness into health. In our day, studies around the placebo effect, which we define as a triggering of our natural self-healing abilities, point us once again to the enormous curative power of expectation. In Epidaurus, after a period of intense preparation focused on a passionate expectation of divine epiphany, the doctor-god would appear to the patient in a dream, providing healing; today the ritually white-coated doctor prescribes an inert procedure that triggers an imagination of cure and heals the patient. Contemporary scientific evidence of this self-healing ability of our bodies is overwhelming, as some of the articles in this book demonstrate.

For several years Steve and I kept on talking, with and without sake, and concluded that a first step was to invite an extraordinary crew of scientists and scholars to the Santa Barbara Pacifica Graduate Institute, of which he is founding president, and have them inform us all. The *Imagination and Medicine* conference, attended by an audience of 250 participants in late April 2007, was the outcome of our musings and our first step toward establishing an Asklepieion for our day.

As you can see from the Table of Contents, the eminent speakers at the conference covered a wide area of scientific scholarship and practice: trauma and healing; studies of the placebo effect; traditional medicine in an African/Western context; psychotherapy and body; the history of integrative medicine and the effects of stress on the physical system; genes and mirror neurons; the traditional place of music as medical therapy (with an entrancing harp performance); dream incubation and Asklepian sanctuaries in antiquity; and the physical architecture of ritual spaces conducive to the healing process.

It was an encompassing experience.

Two months later I travelled to the place where Western medicine began, to the Greek island of Kos, a bit like a pilgrimage.. This island gave birth to Hippocrates, said to have been a descendent of the mythical mortal Asklepios who later became the god of healing. Most doctors swear by Hippocrates.

The harbor town of Kos is a height-of-the-season tourist trap.

I'm walking the streets hardly noticed by the youthful crowd— beautiful in barely suppressed mating frenzy. It is early July, and the heat has cooked the narrow streets with Greek island fragrance. The sun sets a magical orange while the planet Venus, gleaming brightly behind the old harbor, appears in indomitable splendor.

Someone should set this to music.

In its heyday some 2,400 years ago, the island of Kos housed a prosperous family business started around 1000 B.C.E. in the days before Homer, when the mortal Asklepios was said to have had a legendary knack for healing, such that he was able to raise the dead. God of the Underworld Hades protested, so Asklepios lost both his life and his mortality, becoming a god. Since his day his descendents, the Asklepiads, kept his healing magic in the family, until Hippocrates nineteen generations in. Hippocrates, born around 460 B.C.E. as the son and grandson of famous physicians, was a revolutionary. He decided that others should be able to learn his ancestral art as well, and he opened up the Kos medical school to anyone of merit. A nonfamily member with a penchant for healing who wanted to perfect his craft at this renowned medical school needed only to pay a fee and swear an oath, the Hippocratic oath. About two-and-a-half millennia later, doctors still do.

The archeological site of the hospital sanctuary opens at 8 AM, and I take my rented bicycle to ride the twenty minutes to the base of the mountain, having been told by the guidebook that there was no incline. Its author obviously drives a car. I drip upon arrival, not helped by the fact that it is in the mid-30s Centigrade already, close to 90 degrees Fahrenheit.

The site is relatively small, about two ballparks on an incline. Almost everyone who works there is present. The buses with hurried tourists won't come until 9.30 AM.

The sanctuary-cum-school has three levels, the initial level of which, it is explained, contains the open area where the patients were housed, with the necessary latrines. On the middle level stood an altar and small temples for the resident Asklepios and possibly for his mythical father Apollo, plus a no-longer-existent painting of Aphrodite, goddess of love and beauty, which inspired Botticelli's "Primavera," Venus on the half shell, as well as the most famous statue of Aphrodite in all antiquity, by Praxiteles, also gone. Also on the middle level was a place for dream incubation called an *abaton*, about which more later. The upper level offers sweeping panoramas of coastline, glistening blue strait, and bone-dry mountains of the island across. It contains ruins of further hospital rooms as well as a floor plan of the great temple of Asklepios, built a century after the main ones on the second level at a time when the school was obviously grander. Patients would travel from far away to submit to diets, physical exercise, the beauty of the place overlooking the Aegean (much like Santa Barbara), and their intense faith in the healing abilities of the god and his physicians—a faith that today still brings patients to places like Lourdes to be healed of intractable illness.

Local spring-fed healing waters rich in minerals were channeled into the building complex by way of an extensive network of earthen-ware pipes to healing baths, and special diets were recommended, everything you might expect at a spa. Bones were set, operations per-formed, and medicines prescribed as they would be in a contempo-rary hospital.

And then there was one big difference. Something so alien to our current wisdom that it strains our ability to believe the incontrovert-ible historical data, so much so that the guidebook fails to mention it: the patient was dreamed back to health.

The very word "clinic" is derived from the couches in the *abaton*, on which the patient would lie down in the ardent expectation of seeing a representative of Asklepios, or even the god himself, in her dream. Or if you were a bad dreamer you could ask someone else to dream for you.

Western medicine from its inception was aware of the great power of dreaming, not for emotional purposes as used now in some circles ever since the beginning of psychoanalysis but for the treatment of physical illness. For close to a millennium, the people who gave us the foundation of most of Western thought, including science itself as well as its practical applications during the Roman Empire, swore by this method of dream healing.

In walking up to the first level on the monumental staircase, I'm sorry to realize that I feel absolutely nothing. I had been looking for-ward to entering this place of origin where imagination had been strong enough to engender dream-based healing, but I feel bored al-ready. You can't force these matters, so I continue. On the second level is the altar of the god.

The stones seem different: natural, uncarved, unlike the stylized temple from the Roman era standing next to it with its pretty marble columns. They were built five hundred years apart. In these rough stones I can feel the earth from before it was a temple. The altar feels like one to nature itself, very appropriate for a healing sanctuary. Then I notice that I am drawn irresistibly to the gray stone leftovers of a small rectangular Asklepian temple across the way from the nature altar to the god, built at the same time in the early third century B.C.E.

Thus it had been erected within earshot of Hippocrates' life by people who might have known him when they were young. (Hippocrates died around 360 B.C.E. after having lived for a full century.) Behind the remains of a partition, against the outer wall facing the hill, stands what I presume to be a small altar of a shape similar to the temple, made of the same grey stone as the outer wall. I am relieved to see it has not been plundered as almost everything else here has been, probably thanks to its utter simplicity. It looks like a rectangular hollow treasure trove within the center of which is a hole of the same rectangular shape. I sense that maybe here still resides the spirit of place, the genius giving rise to a millennium of healing. On impulse I take my water bottle and spill some of my water into the hole down the hollow box. Then I drink some. As the sun beats down on me I feel part of a strange water-sharing ritual.

Suddenly I have an inexplicable sense in my body that the box is communicating with me.

When I notice these physically felt intuitions, I have learned from my decades as a psychoanalyst to momentarily suspend disbelief, much like a reader of fiction does, and listen carefully. The words I might ascribe to this feeling are: "I want to give you a gift. Look behind this box." I start looking at the back of the box and find a stone of the same color as the box. I assume this must be what the box "intended," and I pocket it.

After some time I leave the temple and walk over to a guard with a green whistle that she uses to restrain impetuous rock climbers and ask her for the *abaton*, the place of the dreamers. She has been looking at me suspiciously, for which I can't blame her in this age of terrorism. Who knows what I poured down the altar. She seems glad to send me in the wrong direction. After a wild goose chase I find the leftovers of the *abaton* right in back of the box that had inspired me to look behind it. In order to enter dreamers' dreams, Asklepios' signal wouldn't have had to travel far. The dreamers were assured good reception.

The *abaton* consists of a large front portico and two rooms behind it, with one or two more rooms in back. From the left backroom, at the far right-hand corner of the high retaining wall that holds the mezzanine terrace above, a stairway leads down five steps into the earth to a triangular opening. I carefully step down towards it. As I look in I see it is a tunnel, about two feet high. Inside are stone slats carefully placed in an inverted v-shape. Where does it lead, this tunnel below the rooms for the dreamers? But for my claustrophobia and fear of things unknown I would enter the narrow triangular aperture reminiscent of womanhood. I photograph it instead, leaning in as far as I dare, camera arm outstretched before me. My flash reveals no end to the triangular tunnel.

I imagine it to reach down to the cave of the snakes who often lived in Greek sanctuaries long before man-made structures were erected, like the great serpent Python of Delphi. The serpent must be the Ancestor of the healing god himself, since one curls up around the staff he carries that still adorns our pharmacies. I shudder and draw back from these stairs to the Underworld.

"I need your help," I mumble to the invisible presence.

According to Hippocrates, the body's resistance can under favorable circumstances eliminate the disease. In his words: "The body's nature (*physis*) is the physician in disease." He suggests that it is the nature of the body to maintain health. The body is its own physician. In saying this, Hippocrates does not deny that the external physician can be of decisive help by attacking the disease head-on through medication or technological procedures—to the contrary. But the physician inside should play a central role in the treatment of illness, according to the founding genius of scientific medicine.

This internal physician can be stimulated by way of the placebo response or through faith healing and the agency of a god. In our day and age, however, many don't believe in divine healers, and many find it unethical to trick patients. We know for a scientific fact that expectation of cure is a significant element of the healing process. Expectation is a specific instance of creative imagination, which brings about what it imagines. Creative imagination has produced all of culture, including science; it brings to life the dreams we have at night as well as those we have for our lives. And in its embodiment as the physician inside it can create health if it is triggered in an effective way.

Here is the problem: we know that creative imagination—in the form of faith in a particular divinity or through the placebo effect— can trigger a self-healing response and can lead to significant medical effects beyond the efficacy of conventional therapies alone. Is it possible to trigger the self-healing response by way of the creative imagination without believing in the authority of any particular god and without being tricked by medical authorities?

Gisela is a physician from Germany who is in remission from colon cancer. Currently she is suffering from severe pains in her kidneys after a bout of high fevers. She is a participant in an incubation trip to Ireland I lead between the *Imagination and Medicine* conference and my journey to Kos. During an incubation journey we visit alien places to trigger unfamiliar dreaming. For the past five days we have followed along the path of the original settlers of Ireland who moved in waves from western to eastern Ireland, as Stone Age immigration followed the great north-south highway of Europe by ship, passing Ireland's western shores. The Irish Stone Age ancestors left behind impressive grave sites, called cairns.

A cairn is a man-made cave construction of large flat boulders ingeniously layered in a roofing structure, the largest of which—the Neolithic cathedral-like marvel of Newgrange—has a high roofing so tight that in its five thousand years of existence it has never experienced a water leak in a country with the highest incidence of rainfall in Europe. These boulders were transported over many miles, before the invention of the wheel, and constructed into cairns over three generations of people whose life expectancy was about thirty years. It took a large number of workers a long time to construct them, more than half a millennium before the great pyramids. Cairns must have been very important to them. When the Irish ancestors began their cairn building in western Ireland, the structures were relatively small, though the great megalithic masterpiece in Newgrange at the bend of the river Boyne in eastern Ireland is gigantic.

When coming upon the first cairn up in the hills overlooking a large section of County Galway, I see our guide go down a little hole. He has told us that we have to crawl on our hands and knees as low as we can for a bit, but then the tunnel will open up in a space large enough for us all to stand. We are a group of ten. Right behind him, Gisela disappears first down the hole. For some reason I believe this passionate Irishman and, after feeling a nauseating wave of claustrophobia, follow the others, holding my breath all the way through the several yards-long stone birth canal. (Without this faith in a guide I will not dare to do the same in Kos a few weeks later.) Indeed it opens up into a cruciform space, a main area and three outcroppings. We are told that when it was first found, the floor was covered with eleven inches of human bones and ashes. We sit here for a while, feeling the weight of the enclosure work upon us.

After we come out, a thunderstorm, quite unusual in these parts, breaks over us, gushing buckets. Drenched, we run back to the cairn, shimmy back in, and see the lightning reflected through the narrow opening. What can I say . . . a Neolithic moment.

The day before Gisela has the dream I'm about to report, we visit the apotheosis of our journey along Ireland's stone circles and cairns, in Newgrange at the bend of the Boyne. The cruciform shape is familiar by now. We walk in through the birth canal into the stone womb with its three outcroppings. After having been inside the small cairns out west, the ceiling of this one feels impossibly high and breathtakingly magnificent. In the right outcropping we see a flat bowl of white stone that must be very heavy but looks so light it might float. I'm standing next to Gisela as we both are absorbed by its artistry. We are guided to look up at the ceiling to see that there has never been fire in this enclosure during the five thousand years of its existence. The only light that ever enters is during the days around winter solstice, when for seventeen minutes this dark womb is penetrated by a ray from the sun that hits a series of sun-like symbols, tracing its trajectory on the very back wall of the final outcropping. This stone temple is a masterful astronomic clock. Awed silence is the only adequate response. I feel a rush of tears and goose bumps.

Gisela dreams:

I participate in a ritual. It happens once a year, and I am the celebrant. Behind me I can hear the mumbling of people. I am much younger than I am now and notice that I am wearing a gown with a long sleeve. In my hands I carry a white shining bone, human or animal. I am a reluctant participant. I have to do this for the others, but I would rather not. I have to enter into the cairn with this bone which gives off light. With great trepidation I do so. It is very hard to cross the threshold. Inside I am alone. It is still. The darkness is lit by the light of the bone which is given off by its very frailty; it is almost immaterial in its refinement. At the far end I see the white flat bowl we saw at Newgrange. On it is a small pile of bones. I will have to drop my bone into the bowl and pick another one. I don't want to. I want to keep my shiny bone. I know that I have to fulfill this ritual act for all the others outside and do it. I select another bone as I drop in mine. Compared to mine it feels very dense. I worry if I have taken the right bone. Then I realize that this has to happen every year so each bone gets refined into such subtlety that it gives off light. If I hadn't made the exchange, my bone would have just disappeared into nothingness. All these bones must be refined, one every year. I walk back with the bone to the people outside.

Through methods I have described elsewhere,* we help Gisela to reexperience the dream and feel this frail light in the bone as it contrasts with the dense heaviness of the stone cairn. After a while Gisela remarks, matter of factly, that the intense pain in her kidneys is gone. She also associates that during her cancer treatment she underwent chemotherapy only for her children—for the others. Alone she wouldn't have done it. I suggest she reenter this dreamed cairn several times a day to treat her cancer, giving her body this dreamed medicine of renewal.

This last instruction may sound flaky to the ears of the rational mind. However, over the many years I have practiced these imagination-based methods, they have proven quite effective on the physical plane.

I propose that this is one way in which creative imagination can trigger the self-healing response without relying on the authority of a god or a doctor. This healing by way of creative imagination is a result of an inspiring immersion in an exceptional, unfamiliar physical environment, like the temple of Asklepios in the medical school of Kos, overlooking the remarkable splendor of the Aegean, or the cairns of Neolithic Ireland. Here the unexpected happens as, like Gisela, we are initiated to the bone into our human frailty, celebrating the mystery of renewal.

This implies that our places of healing be exceptional places, uncommon in beauty and adventure of spirit, unfamiliar and not commonplace. Places that inspire in us a passionate lust for life, encourage the spirit of survival, and seduce our reluctant selves into a love for the frail, painful splendor of being. Temples of healing garlanded with Aphroditic embodiments of beauty, like the ones in Kos whose after-images still reverberate after more than two thousand years. *Yes*, we need the factory-like hospitals constructed around the necessary technology that drives them, but concurrently we also need in-

*Robert Bosnak, *Embodiment: Creative Imagination in Medicine, Art and Travel* (London/New York: Routledge, 2007).

spiring healing sanctuaries to significantly enhance the already-great effects of conventional medicine.

I'm not saying that we have to lead the sick down ancient tunnels crawling on their hands and knees to face the unknown. But do let's follow Hippocrates' advice and aid the physician inside by feeding her with the outlandish riches of creative imagination, so our will to live may body forth health.

Origins

1

Ancient Asklepieia: Institutional Incubation and the Hope of Healing

KIMBERLEY C. PATTON

Medical research begins at last to reveal what indigenous peoples have always known: imagination *is* medicine. There are no illnesses that are not "psychosomatic": what afflicts *soma* always affects *psyche*, and vice versa. The same is true for trauma. For imagination to heal, to act as *pharmakon* and not as poison for the afflicted human body, the sufferer must be an agent. She must be more than one who endures treatments at the hands of others; she must be in alliance with such treatments and enact them. A major therapeutic vehicle in the ancient world was the healing dream. It was the place of encounter between god and patient, sought through incubation. The patient herself was thus not a target of therapy but rather its source, born from within.

THE DREAM DEFICIT

As a nation, we are all tired. Sleeplessness compromises our memory, escalates our stress, and decreases our patience. Our immune systems deteriorate. Urban light pollution robs us even of darkness. We are robbed of sleep's healing interlude by rising in the dark to deal with e-mail, to leave for work before our own children wake up, to beat rush hour. This is the culture of 24/7, of "productivity" and global responsiveness and, perhaps more than anything, of the instantaneous results promised by technology and now expected of most of one's interactions with the outside world. Many Americans live routines of working while triaging the care of small, equally sleepless children, living with constant anxiety about the cost of food, housing, gas, and medicine, or perhaps about whether a husband or wife will arrive home from Iraq on a plane or inside its cargo hold. Insomnia makes aging Americans unwilling keepers of the night watch, the time when regret and loneliness attack with impunity. For homeless Americans, constant vigilance, not rest, is needed to survive the night exposed on the floor of a train station or in a muttering, dangerous shelter.

It is sleep, Shakespeare wrote, that "knits up the ravel'd sleave of care / The death of each day's life, sore labor's bath, / Balm of hurt minds, great nature's second course . . . " (*Macbeth,* Act II, Scene 2). Our raveled sleeves are not knit up; we are, rather, unraveling. We sleep far less than we should. And when we do, it is often with the aid of green moths or other pharmaceuticals that occasionally make people walk, eat, or even drive in their sleep: the night of the living dead.

It stands to reason that we also dream less than we need to. The company that makes one of those medications launched television ads featuring wonderful gatherings of unlikely companions: a beaver, a deep-sea diver in an old-fashioned bell-helmet, and Abraham Lincoln, chatting together in the company lunchroom. The ad's line? "Your dreams miss you." In sleep deprivation, we are no longer nourished by the soul's nocturnal encounters with itself, with the gods, with the wisdom other cultures have found in dreams. As we dream so seldom, our dreams cannot in turn heal us.

In hospitals across America and the rest of the First World, liminal places for transient sufferers who all are on their way somewhere—either back to a kind of health or on to death—the dark is lit by machines that monitor bioelectrical signals. Sleep is very hard to come by in a hospital, a necessarily 24/7 place of overhead lighting where even the less severely ill endure protocols of constant waking for checks or medication throughout the night. Not only night nurses are unable to sleep normally; we actually train our physicians by subjecting them for several years while they are residents to prolonged sleep deprivation. Despite studies that indicate a devastatingly high correspondence between sleep deprivation and clinical errors, provoking reform at some large teaching hospitals, the system remains still resistant to changing this strange and cruel initiation of our healers.

Modern health care delivery thus blocks what in antiquity was believed to be the most powerful therapy of all, especially for the chronically or hopelessly ill: the healing dream. This was notoriously sent by the healing god Asklepios, although there were others: Amphiaraus at Oropus, Trophonius at Lebadeai.[1] The Neoplatonic philosopher Iamblichus wrote of the soul, "And bodies . . . that are diseased, it heals . . . Thus in the Asklepieion illnesses are healed by divine dreams. Through the ordinances of visions that occur at night, the medical art was composed from divinely inspired dreams" (*On the Mysteries of the Egyptians, Chaldeans, and Assyrians* III).

In the ancient Mediterranean and Near East, dreams were entities that did more than embroider waking reality. The Greeks took dreams very seriously and, like the Egyptians, were afraid of the bad ones. Whereas the Egyptians wore amulets to keep away bad dreams, the Greeks thought the evil predicted by dreams could be averted by apotropaic sacrifice, or by telling the dream aloud in the light of the Helios, the sun. In other words, outside of the dream's natural habitat: a way of interrogating the enemy under the lamp, as it were.

Likewise it is not surprising that dreams were taken to be messages from the gods; the Greek verb used, as Carl Alfred Meier points out, is *episkopein*: "to visit." The person does not *have* the dream; the dream *visits* the person, who "sees the god" in that dream. We are as far as possible from the world of the French expression, "*J'ai fait un rêve*."[2] Without the god's appearance (or saint's or Pir's, in modern dreams), the incubated dream is not efficacious, for one cannot be sure of what to do unless one hears it directly from the horse's mouth. Not an "insight," not a personal change or new direction, not a "rethinking": a *god*, who can not only heal in dreams but even beget children or dictate the text of a speech. The famous dreamer and dubious rhetorician Aelius Aristides, whom we will meet later, often wrote his orations *kata ton oneiraton epipnoian*, "according to the inspiration of dreams."

IMAGINATION AND MEDICINE

It has become a truism that Western theories of pathogenesis and corresponding theories of medicine classically define the human organism in biologically materialistic ways. According to the medical model, life, *bios*, can be threatened at cellular and at systemic levels, and that threat should be addressed at those levels. But as different as we are from the ancient Greeks, we are like them in sensing that *bios* is much more than physical; it is also emotional and existential. The wounded or diseased body is a spiritually affected body, a dreaming body. It is a body that generates philosophy. It is also a metaphysical self. This is a reality so obvious as to scarcely need stating. And yet medicine, deliberately and perhaps defensibly setting itself apart from psychology or religious healing, leaves those realms to others, diverging from the lived realities of the patient.

My father, a retired cardiovascular thoracic surgeon who practiced north of Boston, over the years had better patient outcomes and fewer complications than many of his colleagues, a few of them equally superb surgeons of real genius in the operating room. But typically they were explosive or distant individuals with little interest in their patients as human beings. My father, on the other hand, no saint but an indefatigable healer, would spend hours with his patients and their families pre- and post-operatively, discussing their illnesses, their feelings, the meaning of illness in general and, most of all, of the value and beauty of life, even in pain: why it was worth trying to get well after your chest had been sawed open and you felt like death itself.

A hockey player and a railroad worker in college, my macho father also cried a lot, both in front of patients and in the terrible times when he could not save them. Not a religious man, he went into the hospital chapel alone to say thanks to whomever when he "got a tough one through," as he used to say. And he and his colleagues spoke quietly for decades in the halls about "feeding the condor," the imagined bird of prey at the window he first met while a surgical resident at Massachusetts General Hospital in Boston. The bargain worked like this: you asked the carrion-loving condor to eat your old and sickly patient instead of your desperately ill younger patient who had his whole life before him. As your patient's champion and only hope, you bargained with the various gods, animal or otherwise. You were the broker of salvation, and like Asklepios you had many levels to arbitrate, from the cellular to the cosmic.

During the four decades he practiced as a surgeon, my father, a thoroughgoing biological materialist and rationalist, lived in a world of mythical and religious powers with whom he constantly, covertly trafficked. Without reference to fancy holistic theories of illness, since there weren't any during his era of training, he always instinctively treated the whole person, physical and metaphysical. This went beyond a more humane practice of medicine. His surgical outcomes were actually better.

The greater the threat to the self as a physical being indwelled by spirit, by *pneuma*, the greater the corresponding existential issues raised by the illness or trauma will be. Dying persons have the widest penumbra of such issues, as the soul rises up, perhaps in anguish or in ecstasy, seeing the great crossing it must make. The dreams of the dying clearly show this awareness, consciously or not. But chronic illness too has its special metaphysical correlatives, its charged responses and dreams that are unique to each patient. The more hopeless the case, the less likely the patient is to be medically curable, so the less interested the curative physician is likely to be either in her physical symptoms or in her metaphysical ordeal. Yet ironically, the sicker the patient, the more intense all those needs are likely to be.

Thus the indwelled sick body becomes a problematic object from which the doctor senses that she needs to distance herself. Doctors are about intervening, treating, and curing. The corollary reality is that most doctors dislike very ill people, or people for whom there is no clear diagnosis. They dislike those whose ailments are complicated, long-standing, and resistant to medications—people they intuit they cannot help. The truth is that they want to get away from them. As a result, as Jerome Groopman reveals in his *How Doctors Think*, physicians are often unwilling to offer their full attention to the labyrinthine stories or miscellaneous symptoms of their very ill patients, thus perhaps missing telltale clues to a hidden diagnosis or even a previously unimagined cure.[3]

MEDICINE AND FAITH-HEALING IN ANCIENT GREECE

Ancient Greek doctors, the *iatroi* trained in versions of the Hippocratic tradition or in the many (often effective) folk remedies of the day, were no different. In fact, they seemed to have shared policies against treating the incurable, since to lose many patients surely harms medical reputation. There was nevertheless in ancient Greece and later throughout the Greco-Roman world an expansive and for most of us very strange alternative for chronic or apparently hopeless cases of disease or trauma. "The god would take them on himself." It cannot be overemphasized that the clientele of the Asklepieia comprised those for whom no other form of medicine could avail. Those who came were desperate for miracles and grateful for even the smallest relief.

One thank-offering at Epidauros, one that only surfaced in the late nineteenth century, that of Aeschines the Orator, reads, for example, "Having despaired of the skill of mortals, but with every hope in the divine, forsaking Athens, I was healed in three months of a festering wound which I had had on my head for a whole year" (*Inscriptiones Graecae* IV. 255). We are not wrong in ascribing a kind of psychological urgency to the atmosphere of miraculous cures that prevailed there. As Diodorus tells us, "When the art of the physician fails, everybody resorts to incantations and prayers" (Frg. XXX. 43). So also Plutarch, "Those who are ill with chronic diseases and do not succeed by the usual remedies and customary diet, turn to purgatives and amulets and dreams" (*De Facie in Orbe Lunae* 920b). "A religion of emergencies," Arthur Darby Nock called Asklepian worship.[4]

That the presenting needs at the Asklepieia were emergencies by no means necessarily invalidates the historicity of all the cures. We can say that "psychosomatic" cases were of course highly susceptible to cure because such sufferers had every confidence the god would heal them. But was the festering wound of Aeschines, one of the leading *rhetor*s of his day, "all in his head"? Should we completely dismiss the possibility that cures of sickness or traumas also occurred at the shrines of Asklepios and that internal orientation could have also played a significant role in these cures, as it does to this day?

That the psychological self can and does affect the biological self has been powerfully established by Bessel van der Kolk in the field of post-traumatic stress disorder, among many other trajectories of research.[5] As well, placebo studies have moved far beyond the examination of the narrow effect of dummy interventions. The field now also comprises, in the words of Harvard Medical School osteopath and alternative medicine researcher Theodore Kaptchuk, the broad therapeutic effects of "attention, compassionate care, and the modulation of expectations, anxiety, self-awareness, treatment, and setting."[6] In the shrines of Asklepios, the compassionate attention of the god, rendered in the efficacious dream, was reinforced by therapeutic expectations and implemented through treatments ranging from conventional to unorthodox.

There were over a hundred Asklepios shrines, or healing centers, in the ancient world, including the famous ones at Epidauros, Athens, Corinth, and Pergamon in Asia Minor, but they were found as far away as Spain and Algeria. A Roman Asklepieion in Djelma, Algeria, one of the last built before the advent of Christianity in the time of Constantine, provoked an extreme response on the part of Theodosius in the late fourth century; as part of his overall iconoclastic program against pagan worship, the emperor had it completely destroyed.

These were largely outdoor clinics, massively defended not only against intrusion from without but also pollution from within. As the Roman traveler Pausanias wrote of Epidauros in the second century C.E., "The sacred grove of Asclepius is surrounded by bounds on every side. No men die or women give birth within the enclosure; the same rule is observed in the island of Delos."[7] The temple, altar, incubation building, and associated structures, including theaters, athletic stadia, and extensive networks of cisterns, conduits, and healing wells, were completely enclosed, sacred to the god, the *telos* of the pilgrimage of the desperate.

They were places where fountains flowed; snakes and dogs, healing animals, roamed and licked the wounds of the suffering; festivals, processions, and dramatic performances, also held to be therapeutic, were staged in monumental theaters; and artificial lakes allowed regimens of swimming and boating and freezing. The largest Asklepieia also had gymnasia for exercise. The central temples were adorned with inscribed accounts of healing, like that of Aeschines the Orator bearing witness to the god's compassion and power. Pausanias says, "Tablets (*stelai*) stood within the enclosure. Of old, there were more of them: in my time six were left. On these tablets are engraved the names of men and women who were healed by Asclepius, together with the disease from which each suffered, and how he was cured."[8]

The center and heartbeat of Asklepios' cult throughout its lifespan was Epidauros on the Argive peninsula in Greece, the region of the strongholds of many of the Achaean heroes: Mycenae, Tiryns, and Argos. It is a magnificent place, still considered holy ground by the locals. There Asklepios was believed to be buried, and there he was worshipped together with his father Apollo. Excavations have continued there since 1880. The extant sanctuary remains date from the fourth century B.C.E., the time of the expansions of the brilliant architect Polykleitos. The theater, which had the best acoustics in the ancient world, was the locus for the public festivals of the cult every four

years; a penny dropped on the stage of this theater can still be heard
in the topmost row. In the temple sat the famous cult statue of ivory
and gold by the sculptor Thrasymedes (ca. 375 B.C.E.), described in
all its glory five centuries later by Pausanias and often shown on coins:
"The image of Asclepius is half the size of Olympian Zeus at Athens:
it is made of ivory and gold. . . . The god is seated on a throne, grasping a staff, while holding the other hand over the head of a serpent;
and a dog, lying by his side, is also represented."[9]

Were these the predecessors of the exotic clinics, vendors of extreme diets and wild promises of cure, sought by today's Stage IV cancer patients? The difference is that the Asklepieia represented a time-
honored and accepted institution woven not only into the social fabric of ancient Greece but also embraced by more orthodox healers.
The path to the shrine of Asklepios was culturally legitimate. It existed at the far end of the normative spectrum of treatments but was
nonetheless part of that spectrum, not in natural tension with it, as
we might expect (although as Aelius Aristides' *Sacred Tales* shows,
controversy over protocols between temple medicine and *iatroi*
could indeed erupt). If they were at all able, the ill made their way
or were carried to those sanctuaries where they could seek the help
of the god.

From the traditional source "Corpus Hippocratorum," preserved
from medieval texts, we can infer many of the theoretical and empirical aspects of ancient Greek medicine. Hippocratic medicine replaced
the earlier ideas, perhaps Egyptian, of illness as demonic possession,
but envisioned it for the first time as a consequence of nature expressed
in individual physiognomy. Yet there was a lack of skepticism on the
part of ancients toward the Asklepieia as valuable places of genuine
medicine; in particular, an odd (to us) unwillingness on the part of
the Hippocratic doctors to challenge directly the authority of the god.
In fact, both the ancient Greek physicians who practiced in the com-
munities and the priests of the Asklepian sanctuaries considered themselves his followers. On Kos and elsewhere, Hippocratic physicians were
actually called Asklepiadai, or sons of Asklepios.

Hippocrates, who lived from 460–377 B.C.E., was considered an
eighteenth-generation scion of the line of Asklepios and was said to
have received his medical training at the famous Asklepieion on the
isle of Kos. Similarly, prior to becoming the personal physician to the
Roman Emperor Marcus Aurelius, the young Galen studied for four

years as a *therapeutes* at the Pergamene Asklepieion, dissecting animals to learn anatomy.

In sum: in the Greco-Roman world, the lines between empirically-based medicine and what we might call faith healing were not only blurred, they were interwoven or perhaps nonexistent. The determinant for which type of care to seek seemed to be severity of prognosis rather than the legitimacy of one system over another. The pragmatic *iatroi* practiced their own form of imaginative cures, balancing the "humors," trepanning skulls with fatal results, and instigating dangerous bloodlettings; in the shrines, on the other hand, medicine as we understand it was far from absent and may often have brought about real recovery.

THE "BLAMELESS PHYSICIAN" BECOMES A GOD

For close to a thousand years, from around 600 B.C.E.. to 400 C.E.., the archaic through the Hellenistic and Roman periods, Asklepios was one of the most popular deities in antiquity. He was originally a human being, perhaps an historical physician who lived in archaic Greece. The earliest mention of him is found in Homer's *Iliad,* compiled no later than the mid-eighth century B.C.E.., although on textual grounds demonstrably incorporating narratives and traditions as far back as the Bronze Age. In the *Iliad*, Asklepios is mentioned not as a god but simply and reverentially as "the blameless physician (*amunos ieteros, Iliad* 11.518), extremely skilled in the healing arts. Asklepios' two sons Makhaon and Podalirios were themselves combat surgeons for the Greek side during the ten terrible years of the Trojan War.

After his death, Asklepios, dimly-lit by history, apparently began to be honored as a hero and to receive divine honors as the founder of medicine, perhaps with a cult at his birthplace in Trikka (modern Trikala) in Northern Greece, the oldest of his shrines. But he soon acquired a divine genealogy and eventually was worshipped as a god. According to the poets Hesiod (*Catalogues*) and Pindar (*Third Pythian Ode*), he was the son of Apollo, god of light, prophecy, and of healing. His mother was the Trikkaian nymph Koronis, unfaithful to Apollo while he was away at Delphi. When her infidelity was reported to the god by a white raven the god had left to watch her, she was slain by the goddess Artemis. In his wrath, Apollo turned the messenger raven's wings black. In his remorse, Apollo opened his dead lover's body on her pyre to rescue the unborn Asklepios: the oldest European account of a Caesarean birth.[10]

The baby was given to a rather magical creature to raise. Asklepios' foster parent and master teacher in the arts of healing was the wise Cheiron, a centaur: half man, half-horse. Cheiron lived in a remote wilderness cave by the well of Pelethronian, near Mt. Pelion in Magnesia. He knew all the secrets of medicinal herbs and of the treatment of wounds and diseases. His name probably derives from the Greek word for hand (*cheir*). A very old terracotta figure of Cheiron the centaur from the ninth century B.C.E.. was found at Lefkandi on the large Greek island of Euboea, just to the northwest of Athens. The statue has six fingers! As the supreme healer, he was supposed to have had tremendously strong hands, reflecting the close association in the Greek religious imagination between hands and healing. From this idea and the word *cheir* came the ancient Greek words *cheirurgos* and *cheirourgia,* whence of course derive the English words "surgeon" and "surgery."

Joining his wife Epione and twin surgeon sons in the classical period were four daughters, as hailed in an inscription from Erythrai: "Asklepios, the most famous god—i.e., Paian! By him were fathered Makhaon and Podaleirios and Iaso (Healer)—i.e., Paian!—and fair-eyed Aigle (Radiance) and Panakea (Cure-all), children of Epione, along with Hygieia (Health), all-glorious, undefiled."[11] In the Hippocratic Oath, two of the daughters of Asklepios guarantee the physician's oath: "I swear by Apollo the physician, and Asklepios, and Hygiea, and Panakeia, and all the gods and goddesses that, according to my ability and judgment, I will keep this Oath and this stipulation . . ." Their abstract qualities, codified in their names, reflect the divinization of Asklepios himself and his godlike healing powers. His daughter Hygeia is a frequent companion of the god in healing dreams, applying salves and administering drugs.

In Greek and later Roman statues, Asklepios carried or often leaned on a staff (there is a reference to a "taking up of the staff" at his sanctuary at Kos), with a serpent coiled around it. The Mesopotamian god Ninazu (whose name meant "Lord-physician") had a son, Nigizzida, whose symbol was a rod with two intertwined serpents. Why the snake as symbol of health or healing? The connection may go at least as far back as the 5,000-year-old Sumerian epic of Gilgamesh, in which an enterprising snake steals by the pool where Gilgamesh sleeps exhausted and devours the hard-won plant of eternal youth he has gathered from the sea's floor. Ingesting the plant, the snake inherits its life-giving properties. The snake may also have represented rejuvenation because of the shedding and renewal of its skin. Its quick, legless motions seemed miraculous. The ancients ascribed to snakes sharp-sightedness, vigilance, faithful guardianship, and healing knowledge and power. The serpent, like the immortal hero, lived underground.

Especially ascribed to Asklepios was a very specific species, *elaphe longissima*, a southern European snake about five feet in length. It still survives in the valley of the Danube in Germany, where it was introduced by the Romans. It has many of the gentle qualities of the god, rarely striking at man, and is not poisonous. It regularly assisted in cures. In Aristophanes' *Ploutos*, two large serpents rushing from the sanctuary lick the eyes of the blind protagonist, whereupon his sight is instantly restored. In a stone relief found near Athens from the fourth-century B.C.E.., Asklepios himself appears to his devotees in the form of a snake. In a similar relief, the related healer-god Amphiaraos becomes a great snake to lick or suck the poison from the shoulder of the dreamer.

Asklepios' other sacred animal was a dog; along with snakes, dogs were free citizens in his sanctuaries. The dog association is unclear, but an Epidaurean variant of his birth narrative has the god, like Romulus and Remus, being suckled by a wild female dog after his rescue in the wilderness. Like snakes, dogs were regarded as instrumental in healing the sick. In one of the Epidaurean *iamata* seen by Pausanias, "A dog cured a boy from Aegina. He had a growth on the neck. When he had come to the god, one of the sacred dogs healed him—with its tongue—and made him well."[12]

The gods are present everywhere in the Greek universe, in human social and psychological life. As Jean-Pierre Vernant puts it, though, "It is a universe with a hierarchy, a world of different levels, where it is impossible to pass from one to another."[13] During the Trojan War Asklepios' own divine father, Apollo, chastises Poseidon for provoking him, a god, to fight "for the sake of insignificant mortals, who are as leaves are, and now flourish and grow warm with life, and feed on what the ground gives, but then again fade away and are dead" (*Iliad* 21.463-66). This is what the gods actually think of us: we are contemptibly perishable, creatures of the earth who must feed off its fruits before it reclaims us after a brief moment in the sun.

The biography of the "blameless physician" repeatedly signals his mortal origins. Yet perhaps like all physicians, he hated mortality, hated sickness, and fought to save us from both. Legend held that he was killed by Zeus for the offense of raising the dead, particularly, as medical historian James Bailey points out, those condemned to death by the gods, such as the rock-shattered prince Hippolytus—in other words, not only for erasing the adamantine line that separates gods from mortals but also for contravening the will of heaven.[14] Apollodorus attributes to Zeus a jealousy of Asklepios similar to his wrath against Prometheus for the altruistic theft of fire:

> And having become a surgeon, and carried the art to a great pitch, he not only prevented some from dying, but even raised up the dead; for he received from Athena the blood that flowed from the veins of the Gorgon, and while he used the blood that flowed from her left side for the bane of mankind, he used the blood that flowed from her right side for salvation, and by that means he raised the dead . . . But Zeus, fearing that men might acquire the healing art from him and so come to the rescue of each other, smote him with a thunderbolt (*Bibliotheca* III, 10, 3, 5–4, 1).

Asklepios' actions inexcusably threatened to bridge the wide abyss between the undying gods and the ever-terminal ones who worshipped them.

And here we arrive very quickly at the heart of the myth of Asklepios. It is a myth set in that oscillating world between the dying and undying, the world of the hospital, where the boundaries are in flux—except at those awful times when one violates them, as he did. Asklepios' paradoxical connection with both life and death was so strong that his image even appears on an ancient coin found on the tongue of a corpse. The coin was intended to pay Charon, the grim ferryman of the soul, to go across the black river Styx to Hades. But why, if the person was already dead, beyond help, does the coin show the physician? An interesting question. Socrates' last words were "Crito, I owe a cock to Asclepius; will you remember to pay the debt?" (Plato, *Phaedo* 118a). Many believe that Socrates meant that the physician-god had healed him of the disease of living, being nothing but an encumbrance to the philosopher whose soul wanted only to be free in death to return to what was real.

Even as a celestial or quasi-Olympian god, Asklepios retained some of his chthonic or underworld characteristics associated with heroes and with their realm: the earth, home of snakes and genetrix of herbs; it is Earth who sends dreams.[15] The god is invariably showed standing in Greek and later Roman statuary. He is generally bare-chested, a heroic or divine iconographic attribute, and he wears a long cloak. He looks a great deal like the images of Zeus, a bearded, mature man with a broad chest. However, as we noted of his snake, Asklepios is usually portrayed with a far kinder, gentler expression than that of the fierce father of gods and men. He was conceived as supremely beneficent, a kind of tenderly paternal figure. In a classical statue in the Athens National Museum, we find compassion for human suffering etched on his face. He is the great exception among the Greek gods, one who actually cares for mortals and their plight, perhaps because he, as they all would be, was buried in the earth. The cult of Asklepios is correspondingly unique in ancient Greek culture for its high degree of mortal interactivity with the godhead.

There was a notably humanitarian character to both the god and to his cult that was qualitatively different from the harsh, capricious nature of the rest of the Greek gods, all of whom were regarded with fear. Asklepios alone was universally loved and frequently beseeched for help. Because he was empowered to save souls from Hades, he was given the title "Soter," meaning, literally, "savior." In a hymn at Epidauros, he is invoked, "Hail, Lord, Great Saviour, Saviour of the world." In ancient Greek religion, "salvation" had far more of a sense of rescue from real, physical dangers than that of an eternal or spiritual state, although this changed radically by the time of the mystery cults. Early Hellenistic kings like Alexander the Great were called "saviors" of their people because they protected them against invading foreign powers. With this epithet, Asklepios joined the other great intercessory gods of antiquity, among them the goddesses of Eleusis and the twin Dioskouroi, whose mysteries at Samothrace protected those in peril of drowning at sea.

Graciously and in keeping with his palliative nature, Asklepios always arrived at a new place to establish his cult by invitation, never by fiat. The catastrophic plague in Athens in the fifth century may have occasioned his advent to that city and his ratification as a god by the Delphic oracle. The mysterious plague decimated the Athenians, drawn up inside the walls during the long siege of the Peloponnesian War against the Spartans, felling Pericles himself in 429 B.C.. Its horrors were such that the Athenians, an extremely observant and pious people, lost all grasp of their faith, for the gods had failed them. Thucydides gives us a chilling account of that dark time (*The Peloponnesian War* II.47).

A Byzantine tradition, possibly corroborated by classical inscriptional evidence, held that the playwright Sophocles (called in this context Dexion), invited Asklepios to Athens, housed his snake, and set up altars for him.[16] In Athens, Asklepios' two temples were built on (and into) the slopes of the Acropolis, only a stone's throw below the Parthenon and above the theater of Dionysos. The Asklepieion was located at the site of a natural recessed spring, still bubbling about ten meters deep within the hillside. Within this cave the Virgin Mary is still venerated as a healing power, and her spring shrine is decorated with small Greek metal plaques, with feet, arms, and other body parts inscribed on them, just as the thank-offerings to Asklepios were. (The votives from the Asklepieion in Corinth, plaster forms of the body parts the god had healed, fill an entire museum room.)[17]

Asklepios was also gratefully invited to Rome, traveling there in serpentine form. When Rome was troubled by a pestilence in 292 B.C.E., the oracular Sybilline books were consulted and seemed to recommend that the god be summoned immediately to halt the plague. The Roman historian Livy tells us, "Envoys dispatched to bring over the image of Asklepios from Epidauros to Rome fetched away a serpent which had crawled into their ship and in which it was generally believed that the god himself was present. On the serpent's going ashore on the island of the Tiber, a temple was erected there" (Livy 10.47.7). A medallion from the reign of the emperor Antoninus Pius (138–161 C.E..) shows Asklepios in his snake-incarnation, arriving in glory on the prow of the ship at the island in the river. The remains of his new Italian temple-home, which was made in marble in the form of a ship, are still visible at the Isola Tiberi. Later, a Christian church and associated hospital occupied the island shrine where, continuing the Asklepian tradition, slaves and the poor were treated without charge. In Rome, Asklepios became known as Aesculapius and by the second and third centuries was considered the equal of the sun, while Hygieia, now equated with the Roman goddess Salus, was equated with the moon. A Roman Christian sarcophagus from the fourth century C.E. records the name of the deceased as Asklepia.

Asklepios' career as a divine figure and that of Jesus of Nazareth have many similarities; like Asklepios, Jesus was thought to be the son of a god, also possessing supernatural powers of healing. Like Asklepios, Jesus' tomb became a place of cult, and like him Jesus was accorded divine honors after his death. An archaeological discovery at the pool of Bethsaida in the Old City of Jerusalem casts an interesting light on the cultic ties between the two. John 5:2 mentions Bethsaida, in whose five porticoes lay "a multitude of invalids, blind, lame and paralyzed." The sick waited for the angel of the Lord, who troubled the water at "certain seasons," with a tonic effect on whoever was lowered into the pool immediately afterward. This is where John tells us that Jesus bade a man who had been ill for thirty-eight years, helpless and motionless poolside, to "rise, take up your pallet, and walk."

Excavations of an earlier shrine over which the Christian basilica was built revealed a stone votive foot from Hadrianic times with a Greek inscription bearing the name of the Roman dedicator, a woman. In Hellenistic Palestine in Jesus' time, it may well have been the case that so many sick people lay near the pool because, like so many healing fountains and springs, it was sacred to Asklepios.

"The Curing of Human Suffering": The Dream Encounter

As Patricia Cox Miller writes of dreams in late Western antiquity: "As a discourse of signs, dreams took ancient dreamers . . . deeply into the very intimate areas of body and emotion. It would be difficult, indeed, to overestimate the role played by dreams in the curing of human suffering."[18]

What did the curing of human suffering mean in the cult of Asklepios? This question is a crucial one, and its answer is far from obvious. I mentioned earlier doctors' instinctive avoidance of hope-lessly ill people. The Asklepieia offered such chronic sufferers imme-diate attention and direct consultation, even though there can be no doubt that many, probably the majority, left uncured. This consulta-tion, the god's prescriptions, and oftentimes the healing itself in the form of a dreamed surgery, a supernatural phlebotomy, or the appli-cation of a salve or custom-mixed drug, took place through dreams dreamt in consecrated spaces and superintended by ritual experts. The encounter was, above all else, direct and unmediated. Celsus, the second century C.E. polemicist against Christianity, wrote, "Many men have seen Asklepios, not merely a vision of him, but he him-self as he heals diseases, dispenses benefits, and predicts the fu-ture" (*The True Word*).

The dream was incubated— hatched, as it were—at a therapeu-tic site, the *abaton*, the place of no-walking, usually close by the god's own temple. In the classical period, preparations were relatively simple:

purification in water, using the extensive system of sacred springs and wells within the walls, and sacrifices, some bloodless; by the Roman period, more elaborate torchlight processions may have developed. Porphyry (*On Abstinence* II, 19) and Clement of Alexandria (*Stromateis* 5.1.13) repeat the inscription over the entrance to Epidaurus, "Pure must be he who enters the fragrant temple; purity means to think nothing but holy thoughts."[19] This is a sublimation, however, of an earlier, older prohibition, which was very much about physical purity and lack of contamination.

The suppliant to Asklepios was never alone. She was cared for from the outset of her visit by attendants, who showed her where to sleep, on a *kline* (couch) or directly upon the floor. She slept nearby others who sought healing and help. She slept nearby the god in order to be tended by him. The dream was the consulting room in which one encountered the god-physician. It was itself the theater of healing. Asklepios visited the individual sufferer privately and often immediately undertook to alleviate her symptoms with his own hands. Alternatively he prescribed regimens to be undertaken within the sanctuary confines, as long as the therapies took, to make things better. Thus the incubated dream was also the centerpiece of a concentric series of circles that encompassed both dreaming and waking states.

Aelius Aristides, a hypochondriac orator from second century B.C.E. Pergamon in Asia Minor,[20] presents in his *Sacred Tales* one of the most striking accounts of a dream epiphany and of the magnetic, tender shock it induced in the dreamer.

> For there was a seeming, as it were, to touch him and to perceive that he himself had come, and to be between sleep and waking, and to wish to look up and to be in anguish that he might depart too soon, and to strain the ears and to hear some things as in a dream, some as in a waking state. Hair stood straight, and there were tears of joy, and the pride of one's heart was inoffensive. And what man could describe these things in words? If any man has been initiated, he knows and understands.[21]

The god's coming was the fulcrum of all the ritual activity preceding it and all that would ensue afterwards. It was an iconic encounter. It was the goal of the sought dream. Interestingly, by the time of Aristides, whose case Galen references in his writings, vicarious therapeutic dreaming was possible. One could dream healing dreams for another: In dreams of late summer in 148 C.E., Aristides not only begs the god to save his foster father Zosimus but dreams vicariously of cures for him (Behr sets dream narratives in italics, waking experience in Roman):

> *When the God appeared, I grasped his head with my two hands in turn, and having grasped him, I entreated him to save Zosimus for me. . . . The God refused. For the third time I grasped him and tried to persuade him to assent. He neither refused nor assented, but held his head steady, and told me certain phrases, which it is proper to say in such circumstances since they are efficacious.* And while I remember these, I do not think that I should reveal these purposelessly.

> *But he said that when these were recited, it would suffice. One of them was*—Take care!

> What happened to him after this? First of all Zosimus recovered beyond expectation from that disease, being purged with barley gruel and lentils, as the God foretold to me on his behalf, and next he lived four months besides. So we met one another and feasted together, since the God also helped me much, continuously and strangely.[22]

Similarly, another foster father, Neritus, dreams later of the necessary replacement of all of Aristides's bones and nerves. But, so related Neritus to Aristides, they were not simply to be replaced, new for old. Instead, there had to be a "certain change of those existing, and thus there was need of a great and strange correction." The god tells the dreamer that this can be accomplished through the ingestion thrice daily of unsalted olive oil.[23] Pergamene temple warden Philadelphus dreams of Aristides drinking wormwood diluted with vinegar, after a vision of him standing in the Sacred Theater surrounded by men in white, "hymning the God."[24] As Aristides himself had dreamed the same dream about the drink, he reingests it copiously, to great salutary effect.

In these ancient accounts, Asklepios the dream-surgeon, at times taking the form of a snake or a dog, healed the afflicted organ during the dream or else prescribed therapeutic regimens to be undertaken in the confines of the sanctuary after the dreamer awoke. In dreams he does predictable things, like removing abscesses or extracting embedded weapons. He also does weird things, surreal things, godlike things. He cuts open an abdomen to remove an abscess in one dream, covering the floor of the *abaton* with blood, or excises an eyeball and inserts drugs into the open socket. He severs a head and reattaches it.

Upon waking, unlike in our modern hospitals although not unlike in our modern hospices, the sufferer found the healing environment of the dream reinforced by the sanctuary in which it was dreamed. The sanctuary or *temenos,* but especially the Asklepieion, was a place "set apart," literally "cut apart" (from *temnein,* "to cut") from normal collective life. With rare exception (such as the god's famous healing shrine on the Isola Tiberi in the middle of the putrid river running through Rome), Asklepieia were established in places of great natural beauty, far beyond the polis with its bustling agora and distracting life of constant transaction. The dream would have been retold to cult attendants and fellow patients as an interior event of great value with exterior consequences. The patient was offered interpretation of her dream at once. Whatever length of time divine prescriptions required, she was free to stay until she was well. It scarcely needs mention that this also sharply deviates from the managed care of today, which often ejects sick people back to the undifferentiated chaos of secular life before they are ready to leave the liminal space of the hospital.

Certainly cures at these shrines included recognizably contemporary holistic therapies such as rest, exercise, psychology, bathing, and engagement in music and drama. But they also included bizarre measures such as the eating of figs mixed with ashes from the god's altar, naked marathons in freezing rain, abstinence from bathing for weeks, and bodily suspension upside down for long periods of time. As we have said, dream cures often entailed graphic accounts, including radical surgery, challenging any facile assumption of sublimation. An entire set of surgical instruments was excavated at Epidauros, perhaps to enact a surgery stipulated in an incubated dream, *pace* assertions such as Meier's: "Nor were there any physicians in the sacred precinct and no medical therapy of any kind."[25] This we cannot say with certainty; indeed, the evidence contravenes.

Often the divine prognosis or even the ailment itself may seem to us to be so fantastic as to be unintelligible, locked in the foreign country that is the past. A number of inscriptions of this kind, called *iamata,* survive from the classical period, which were dictated by recovered patients to sanctuary scribes, most likely priests. These describe in first-person the original illness or injury and its miraculous cure at the

Asklepieia. The most famous and complete were the six Pausanias saw at Epidauros; two of the six were excavated, along with fragments of two others.

They are encyclopedic, listing multiple stories of complaints and cures. From Stele I: "Cleinatas of Thebes with the lice. He came with a great number of lice on his body, slept in the Temple, and sees a vision. It seems to him that the god stripped him and made him stand upright, naked, and with a broom brushed the lice from off his body. When day came he left the Temple well" (I. 28).

Gorgias of Heracleia was in a worse way: "Gorgias of Heracleia with pus. In a battle he had been wounded by an arrow so badly that he filled sixty-seven basins with pus. While sleeping in the Temple he saw a vision. It seemed to him the god extracted the arrow point from his lung. When day came he walked out well, holding the point of the arrow in his hands" (I. 30).

And some are beyond the pale:

> Aristagora of Troezen. She had a tapeworm in her belly, and she slept in the Temple of Asclepius at Troezen and saw a dream. It seemed to her that the sons of the god, while he was not present but away in Epidaurus, cut off her head, but, being unable to put it back again, they sent a messenger to Asclepius asking him to come. Meanwhile day breaks and the priest clearly sees her head cut off from her body. When night approached, Aristagora had a vision. It seemed to her the god had come from Epidaurus and fastened her head on to her neck. Then he cut open her belly, took a tapeworm out, and stitched her up again. And after that she became well (I. 23).[26]

Ancient incubations, no matter how elaborated their symbolic expression, usually produced very practical dream recommendations or predictions, and this was most markedly true in the case of dream cures. However these were enacted, they were not merely symbolic. Mystery continues to surround what went on in these centers, but we know a great deal about what people believed went on. The primary goal of such epiphanies was, in fact, healing—not, as might be easier for the postmodern mind to digest, spiritual transformation, but clinical cure—in which the god who came in the dream was an expert physician whose expertise far outstripped that of any mortal.

So the ancient writer Diogenes Laertius distinguishes: "Phoebus Apollo gave to mortals Asclepius and Plato, the one to save their souls, the other to save their bodies" (*Vita Philosophorum* 3.5).[27] Rather than revealing the healing dream as a sublimated entity whose efficacy was purely psychological or spiritual, centuries of evidence from antiquity instead repeatedly attest to literal cures of dire physical illnesses or traumas. Sometimes these were partial or temporary, and relapses sent the sufferers back to Asklepios. Sometimes, or so the claims ran, they were total and permanent.

The sufferers, relieved of the disease or affliction that had been tormenting them, the suppurating wound or the pregnancy gestating for years, saw the god doing things to their dream bodies. But their waking bodies walked out of the sanctuary holding the long-buried arrow point, holding the once-trapped, overdue baby.

Payment was always due: money if possible, although the poor were subsidized. Offerings and inscriptions told the world what had happened in the dream and its real-life consequences. The grateful patient of Asklepios who successfully implemented his advice dedicated *iatra* or *sostra*, thank-offerings, according to his wealth. These could take, among other things, the form of sacrificed cock (as in Socrates' final words to Crito), a composed paean, the erection of a stone stele with an account of the incubation and its aftermath, or a sculpted image of the healed body part to show the world what the god had done for the suppliant in his dreams. Cases of godsent relapse in the event of tardy payment are known.[28] Again, the bottom line was actual cure, undertaken or envisioned in the therapeutic dream in graphic detail.

The aftermath of an intense or prolonged incubation could be a degree of possession by or absorption into the deity; after the incubation, if it produces the desired dream of the god, one's life is no longer entirely one's own. It is as though the prolonged contact through dreams with the holy place, and thus with the god that lives there, has blurred the edges of the distinct and socially defended personality; the god has infested the dreamer. This is, understandably, especially true of healing dreams, and the worse the illness or wound, the truer it is. There can be said to be a kind of fusion of the smaller self with the larger, and this might even be asserted without psychoanalytic overtones. That fusion can be forged by gratitude alone, and it is a result of an invasion of the personal world of one's dreams by the transpersonal godhead.

Later these extreme cases might stay at the healing shrine and become permanent fixtures, dream "hangers-on"; in Hellenistic Greek cultures, they were called *katochoi*, literally, "voluntary prisoners," such as the notorious and prolific Aelius Aristides, who took up residence at the Asklepieion at Pergamon intermittently for a total of twelve years. This condition is not a pathology separate from that of a normal seeker of dreams at the shrine. Rather, it simply represents a more extreme existential condition and behavior on the spectrum of incubation; that spectrum inevitably mandates identification with the god who *dreams through* and thus *into* the sufferer. One belongs to the goddess by dint of having dreamed her; this is made manifest by those who remain at the incubation shrine instead of going home.[29]

Although they are no more, Asklepieia are linked phenomenologically to other incubation sites and traditions throughout the world, including those still used in present time. Physical healing through dreams continues in the Eastern Orthodox Church in great churches at Cyprus, Tinos, and Constantinople, and in small churches everywhere. The Church at Constantinople in particular was active as a center of healing dreams in the name of Roman soldier-martyrs of the pre-Constantinian period—twin physicians, The Holy Unmercenaries Ss. Cosmas and Damian—since Byzantine times; it seems however to have been built on a classical incubation shrine sacred to the healing god-twins, the Dioskouroi.

An Orthodox nun, Aemiliane, living in a women's monastery near Meteora, in northern Greece, reported to my husband in 2002 an account of miraculous dream healing. Another nun's (Miriam's) grandfather, suffering from gangrene, traveled to the Church of Ss. Cosmas and Damian in Trikala, about twenty minutes from Meteora, and slept there overnight. He was healed in a dream and continued to visit the church, which was not his own parish, making the trip on foot every Sunday for the rest of his life to express his gratitude to the saints, known for their medical skill and their refusal to accept payment for their work.

Note that the suffering man lay down to sleep in a church, a shrine, to which he had to travel on foot and with which he had no ordinary link other than previous traditions of incubation healings that took place there. He was healed of gangrene, a notoriously serious condition that will eat up a limb and destroy it, and one that is perfectly in keeping with the kind of gross, aversion-causing ailment that seems so characteristic of the things people brought to Asklepios. Lying down to spend the night in the church alone, the old man was visited in a dream by the saint-physicians, who were both doctors, just as the god Asklepios began his career in Homer's *Iliad* as a mortal solider. He was healed literally overnight, responding with a regular, arduous pilgrimage every week. The trip to this parish was his testimony, his inscription, his thank-offering (*charisterion*), showing the world what happened in his dream.

EVALUATING ASKLEPIAN CLAIMS OF CURE

At least three major ways of interpreting this evidence emerge in the literature. The first, one of thorough skepticism, sees the cultus and its complexes as part of a self-reinforcing and self-justifying collective, a crystalline illustration of the social theory of Durkheim or of Freud's view of religion as compensatory illusion. As the scholar C. A. Behr, translator of the *Sacred Tales* of Aelius Aristides, writes, "These cures do not really convey the impression of reality, and the Epidaurean Tablets seem due to the fraudulent desire of that Temple's priesthood to magnify the power of their God."[30] At best, this view has it, the Asklepian approach offered a kind of culturally supported panacea.

Two years ago, I attended grand rounds in the oncology department at Massachusetts General Hospital in Boston with my brother, a department administrator there. The morning's topic was recent data from studies done in two major hospitals in different parts of the country indicating the strong desire of a large number of patients to have their spiritual needs addressed during their hospital stay; a surprising percentage even said they would like their physician to pray for or with them. The presenter, a social worker in the oncology unit with strong research interests in religion and medicine, reminded the department of the original meaning of *hospital* ("guest-house") and of the fact that since the time of the Dark Ages, the very ill sought refuge at monasteries and were received as guests along with healthy pilgrims. One and all, they were cared for without charge in the name of Christian hospitality. During the Q & A, one oncologist expressed irate impatience with the idea that he should divert any of his clinical time to facilitate what he called "some coping mechanism."

So the first approach argues that no real cures took place at the Asklepieia other than those that would have occurred anyway. At best, these shrines offered an elaborate coping mechanism, but unlike today's alternative spa-clinics in Mexico or Switzerland, these were culturally sanctioned and, for many, located right up the road.

The second approach to ancient claims of healing lifts up the soul, rather than the body, as the true object of healing in the cult of Asklepios. Jungian analyst and classicist Carl Alfred Meier developed this approach, inspired by the prominent place of the arts, music, and theater in larger Asklepieia such as Epidaurus:

> It can be said that what actually was provided for in these clin-ics of antiquity was the *cura animae* and that it really was a cult of the psyche, which itself should be the object of true therapy. The ensemble of water, snakes, trees, art, and music, theater and a chthonic cult whose acme came about at night in a dream seems to explain a good deal of these miraculous effects. It is certainly more inclusive than what is offered at healing places these days whether at a University clinic or at Lourdes.[31]

Along these lines, Dr. Michael Kearney's work in palliative care employs an Asklepian approach that attends with focused compassion not only to the physical needs but also to the dreams and psychologi-cal issues of the dying. In *A Place of Healing*, Kearney has shown through case studies how the holistic approach of the Asklepieion can be applied brilliantly.[32] The patient's dream work and journal keep-ing, in the matrix of the physician's focused and sustained attention, may reveal the soul's deepest agenda. From bitterness, denial and, above all, despair, the ordeal of dying can be reoriented to a resolu-tion of unfinished issues, a healing of relationships, and sometimes a yearned-for rapprochement with the divine. Hence the emergence, even at the eleventh hour, of the spiritual self.

That the dying often dream prophetic or "big" dreams is a staple of myth and fairytale but is also realized in the pastoral clinical work of hospice care. Scholar of religious dreams in religion Kelly Bulkeley and his mother Reverend Patricia Bulkeley, a hospice chaplain, have published a series of extraordinary pre-death dreams and visions in their book *Dreaming Beyond Death*.[33] The following befell Suzanne, an elderly patient in the final stages of a terminal disease:

> One morning she told her doctor she had just awakened from a dream: *She sees a candle on the windowsill of the hospital room and finds that the candle suddenly goes out. Fear and anxiety ensue*

as the darkness envelops her. Suddenly, the candle lights on the other
side of the window and she awakens. That same day Suzanne died,
"completely at peace."[34]

Note that Suzanne told her doctor this dream, and the doctor felt that
it was significant enough to record, to remember.

The second approach is thus largely uninterested in the veracity
of the physical healings reported in the ancient evidence. It dwells
instead on the healing of the soul that clearly also took place at the
Asklepieia through use of water, through music and drama, through
exercise and the practice of beauty, but most of all through focused
attention to the dreams and total situation of the sufferer. She left
feeling cared for by the god and by those in his service. What greater
therapy could there be? Spiritual transformation is the main interest
of the second approach, as evidenced by one character created by the
Hellenistic playwright Menander:

> Believe me, men, I had been dead during all the years of life
> that I was alive . . . The beautiful, the good, the holy, the evil
> were all the same to me; such, it seems, was the darkness that
> formerly enveloped my understanding and concealed and hid
> from me all these things. But now I have come here, I have
> become alive again for all the rest of my life, as if I had lain down
> in the temple of Asklepios and been saved. I walk, I talk, I think.
> This sun, so great, so beautiful, I have now discovered, men for
> the first time; now today I see under the clear sky you, the air,
> the acropolis, the theater (*Papyrus Didotiana*, b, 1–15).[35]

How easily could this have been written by a recovering sufferer of
clinical depression or by one who has narrowly escaped death? The
second approach, in other words, champions the way in which human beings can be reoriented at the shrines of Asklepios and leave "well"
in a sense that transcends literal cure.

The third approach admits that some real cures and healings did
take place at these shrines but argues that they did so not through
any real practice of medicine but rather as a result of autosuggestion
and secondary elaboration. Echoing many others, Behr writes:

> The mechanism lay in the dreamer's knowledge of medicine and
> in autosuggestion as his subconscious alternately conjured up
> reasonable and fantastic remedies. The expectancy of the
> incubants and their frequent discussions about cures and medi-

cine would channel their dreams by means of secondary elaboration, if this were needed, into real or pseudo-medical forms.[36]

Unlike the Epidaurean testimonies, Aelius Aristides' account of
his numerous visits to the Pergamene shrine reveals sharp tensions
between conventional medicine and the bizarre dream cures indicated
by the god, with whom he had a lifelong, intimate relationship. To
the horror of most conventional doctors, Aristides is given numerous
phlebotomies, or made to walk for miles in the blistering sun or freezing
cold in a weakened state. His faithful physician Theodotus alone carries out the god's orders, but often with barely concealed distress.

The third take on these reported cures is also championed in the
conclusions of Ludwig and Emma Edelstein, the husband-and-wife
team who collected ancient testimonies in their two-volume work
Asklepios and offered an extensive analysis of what they call "temple
medicine." They first note that the dreams themselves, the epiphanies of the gods, can be explained by the preexisting orientation of
the patients, who were, it must be remembered, also pilgrims:

> Coming in quest of the god's help, excited by the long journey
> which sometimes they had undertaken for this selfsame pur-
> pose, preoccupied with their suffering as they must have been,
> having seen the sights of the sanctuary and having stayed in
> these surroundings at least for a number of hours, having read
> the tablets on which the reports on portentous dreams and suc-
> cessful cures were inscribed—how could the supplicants fail to
> dream as they did?[37]

The Edelsteins note that while certain miracle cures sound irrational, others manifest an aura of scientific rationality. The dream-
surgeon Asklepios performs incisions with instruments, for example;
he uses cupping glasses; he prescribes drugs (some are known
pharmaka, others of his own invention). Dream cures, the Edelsteins
say, must be taken as "historical facts." On the one hand, they suggest spontaneous healings in the case of hysterical blindness, or the
ejection of kidney stones in urine or nocturnal emission; or the role of
shock itself. On the other hand, they equivocate: "Even if the patients
of Asclepius only dreamed, even if their cures were only a rationaliza-
tion of what they believed they had seen, it is not astonishing that
the Asclepieia could claim so many real healings."[38]

This third line of response dwells very heavily on the orientation
and existing knowledge of the patient himself. In other words, the

cures dreamed are themselves cultural artifacts or, in the words of E. R. Dodds, "culture pattern dreams,"[39] undivorced from the medicine of the day or from quotidian experience. The Edelsteins and others have noted the way that the medical content of Asklepian dreams tended to evolve across time as cures and practices also evolved; the dreams became more sophisticated as the treatment of trauma and disease also evolved in the waking world. This would not necessarily have diminished their effectiveness, a subtlety often lost on those—and they are legion—who hold that mere demonstrability of social context of any metaphysically-based claim *de facto* negates its validity.

Above all else, there was the powerful expectation that the god would cure; that coming to him would work. Time and again in the testimonies Asklepios asks the patient to trust him completely, expressing his disdain for cowards. "The patient's confidence, then, was a factor which came into play in human medicine no less than in divine, the only distinctive feature of Asklepios' healings being that they eclipsed all human hopes and expectations."[40] The placebo effect, once maligned as evidence of the human capacity for self-delusion, has been rehabilitated over the past decade by Theodore Kaptchuk[41] and through ongoing clinical research at Columbia University by Tor Wager and others: placebo is real, with a genesis in the deep brain rather than just resulting from psychological disposition.[42] Furthermore, it produces real, clinically measurable effects, effects that may potentially extend beyond the limits of pain's metrics.

The mind-body connection is largely beyond our present ability to appreciate, although we are beginning to acknowledge its indicators: the work of Esther Sternberg and others, for example, highlights quantifiable phenomena such as the effects of neurologically mediated stress on the immune system at the cellular level.[43] Yet we all swim in anecdotal evidence. How the mother refused to die until the last child showed up at her bedside. How a friend eschewed interferon and stopped the march of Hepatitis C through her liver with yoga and acupuncture instead, essentially refusing to fall ill. How it works is unclear, but the hope and expectation of healing is clearly not an insignificant feature in many cases of "real" cure. "Even though their drugs were curious and their regimens paradoxical, Asclepian dreams functioned by making the healing process palpable. To the ill, dreams presented striking visual images, often in the form of a visitation by the god Asclepius himself, and these images redirected the attention of the dreamer away from disease and toward cure." Through the dream, one was reoriented: "toward one's conscience, toward one's future, toward one's body."[44]

Indeed, if the Asklepieia really worked in some cases to effect real cures, then the potential of human dreaming must acquire new and deeper dimensions. The godsent (*theopemptos*) dream would emerge as part of a therapeutic alliance, mostly now obscure to us. The alliance consisted of existing medical knowledge, collective healing environments, and placebo response. All these were recombined and deployed through the channels of ritual. Such ritual channels would have been designed, as anthropologist Talal Asad asserts, to produce believing bodies, persons physically and mentally disposed through religious practices toward particular orientations[45]—in this case, the healing power of the compassionate physician. That such ritually inscribed bodies could actually get well—overcoming real pathologies at the Asklepieia—is a possibility we have, up till now, been largely unwilling to concede.

Present Realities: The Hope of Healing

Can the heritage of Asklepios offer anything to our mainstream models of disease or trauma and their treatment? As I have tried to suggest, honest confrontation with the historical evidence raises questions, among them that of the extent to which physical illness can be ameliorated through integrative (psychosomatic) approaches. If the entire person, comprising interrelated physical and metaphysical selves, is carefully attended to—dreams and all—is there still potential, as there may have been at Epidauros and elsewhere, for a better therapeutic outcome? And is an approach that honors both body and soul—honors the sufferer as a *hospes*, a guest—now lost and unrecoverable, since unanchored from its original context?

The hopeless cases, the chronically ill, have always needed compassionate and sustained *attention*. The ancient Greeks knew this and created ritual spaces for the giving of such attention. Attention to the one who is afflicted, which Simone Weil has called "a very rare and difficult thing," has been made even more difficult by managed care. Groopman notes that "most patients are gripped by fear and anxiety; some also carry a sense of shame about their disease. *But a doctor gives more than psychological relief by responding empathetically to a patient.*"[46] Groopman cites Debra Roter, a health policy professor at Johns

Hopkins, who together with Judith Hall at Northeastern University studies medical communication. Roter observes that in addition to asking open-ended questions about a patient's symptoms:

> The physician should respond to the patient's emotions . . . the patient does not want to appear stupid or waste the doctor's time. Even if the doctor asks the right questions, the patient may not be forthcoming because of his emotional state. The goal of a physician is to get to the story, and to do so he has to understand the patient's emotions.

In *The Illness Narratives,* Arthur Kleinman similarly warns that when a patient's story is truncated and medicalized, it is thus often diminished in clinical value *because of ignoring or excluding her description of the effects of the disease on her life and existential situation.*[46] By restoring the patient's full narrative, the doctor restores meaning to the sufferer and is furthermore in a better position overall to treat the problem. The doctor can become a healer: an archetypal role reserved in the ancient Greek world for the gods alone.

Our modern hospitals are no longer located outside of cities or towns; such remoteness is not a priority. Our very sick are far from sleeping on the earth, and they surely do not sleep side by side, breathing in rhythm. Sleep—deep, restorative sleep—is almost unattainable in modern hospitals. Because most, although not all, dreams occur during REM sleep, healing dreams there are all but impossible. Even if they do occur, who is there to interpret them? Music, drama, art, sacred animals: these could not be further from our clinical environments. Running water, therapeutic baths, or healing fountains are nowhere to be found. The ancient possibility of extended stays is annihilated by managed care, which aims at producing markers of recovery only just sufficient enough to stop payment for the treatment and send the patient home. We can scarcely forget the ways that the poor, the uninsured, often the most grievously prone to chronic illness, cannot receive adequate care in many American hospitals.

Most crucially, we have lost a wholehearted belief in the god who can heal. Perhaps he can be summoned from our dreams, if there is still a way to recover them.

NOTES

[1] See the discussion of the therapeutic power ascribed to dreams in antiquity in Chapter 4, "Dreams and Therapy," of Patricia Cox Miller's revelatory study *Dreams in Late Antiquity: Studies in the Imagination of a Culture* (Princeton, NJ: Princeton University Press, 1994). On the special identity of dreamers, the sick, and the founders of sanctuaries, see Folkert van Straten, "Images of Gods and Men in a Changing Society: Self-identity in Hellenistic Religion," in *Images and Ideologies: Self-definition in the Hellenistic World*, ed. Anthony W. Bulloch, Erich S. Gruen, A. A. Long, and Andrew Stewart (Berkeley: Univ. of California Press, 1993), 248–265, esp. 258–259.

[2] The notion of dreams as the product of the dreamer is known elsewhere, as in Indian thought, although in the *Brhadahanyaka Upanisad* the dreamer *creates* an interior reality from the stuff of his outer reality: " . . . there are no ponds, lotus-pools, or flowing streams there; but he emits ponds, lotus-pools, and flowing streams. For he is the Maker" (*Brhadahanyaka Upanisad* 4. 3. 9–10, translated and discussed by Wendy Doniger [O'Flaherty] in *Dreams, Illusions, and Other Realities* [Chicago: University of Chicago Press, 1984], 16). As Doniger points out, however, this ontology makes the dreamed world no less real. In fact, traditionally, the dreamed world is *more* real than the waking one. In culturally inflected ways, this also describes the ancient Greek view.

[3] Jerome Groopman, *How Doctors Think* (Boston: Houghton Mifflin, 2007), esp. Introduction.

[4] Arthur Darby Nock, review of Emma Edelstein and Ludwig Edelstein, *Asclepius: Collection and Interpretation of the Testimonies*, Volumes I and II (Baltimore: Johns Hopkins Univ. Press, 1945), in *Classical Philology* 45 (1950): 48.

[5] E.g., among many other works, Bessel A. van der Kolk, "The Body Keeps the Score: Approaches to the Psychobiology of Posttraumatic Stress Disorder," in *Traumatic Stress: The Effects of Overwhelming Experience on Mind, Body, and Society*, ed. Bessel A. van der Kolk, Alexander C. McFarlane, and Lars Weisaeth (New York: Guilford Press, 1996); "The Psychobiology of Posttraumatic Stress Disorder," *Journal of Clinical Psychiatry* 58 (1997): 16–24.

[6] T. J. Kaptchuk, "The Placebo Effect in Alternative Medicine: Can the Performance of a Healing Ritual Have Clinical Significance?" *Annals of Internal Medicine* 136 (11) (June 4, 2002): 817.

[7] Pausanias, *Descriptio Graecae* II, 27, 1; Edelstein and Edelstein, *Asclepius* [1998 ed.] I, T. 739: 383. Along these lines, indicating the severe extent to which these purity laws were applied and over how many centuries, later in the same account Pausanias notes the compassion of the Roman senator Antoninus of his day: "The Epidaurians about the sanctuary were in great distress, because their women were not allowed to bring forth under shelter, and their sick were obliged to die under

the open sky. To remedy the inconvenience he provided a building where a man may die and a woman may give birth to her child without sin." Author's note on "remedy the inconvenience"[!]: The Edelsteins' translation of *epanorthoumenos* is remarkable; the ancient Greek has the sense of rectifying a wrong or amending a situation. That the Epidaurians were said by Pausanias to have been in "great distress" gives a truer picture of what it must have been like to be forced to give birth or die out in the elements: agony, not inconvenience.

⁸ Ibid. 27, 3; *Asclepius* I, T. 739: 381–385.

⁹ Ibid. 27, 2; *Asclepius* I, T. 739: 383.

¹⁰ The Epidaurian version predictably made Epidaurus the birthplace of Asklepios, where the baby was nurtured by a goat and a dog (reflected in the prohibition against goat sacrifices to the god, and the ubiquity of sacred dogs in his cult). The site of the famous sanctuary of Asklepios at Epidaurus, dating around 500 B.C.E., was previously the focus of a cult of Apollo Maleatas dating back to the Bronze Age.

¹¹ Inscription from Erythrai, *Greek Lyric V: The New School of Poetry and Anonymous Songs and Hymns,* ed. and trans. David A. Campbell (Cambridge: Harvard University Press, 1993). Frag. 939.

¹² Edelstein and Edelstein, *Asclepius* I, T. 423 (26): 234.

¹³ Jean-Pierre Vernant, *Myth et Société en Grèce Ancienne* (Paris, ed. La Découverte, 1974, 1992): 104.

¹⁴ James E. Bailey, "Asklepios: Ancient Hero of Medical Caring," *Annals of Internal Medicine* 124, 2 (15 January 1996): 257–263.

¹⁵ The temple with its cult statue honored Asklepios as a god, but like Herakles, as one who had died and been promoted to divine honors, he had a dual nature. He was also a hero. Heroes were thought to live underground after death, joining the infernal powers. Asklepios' chthonic personality as a dead and therefore energetic hero may or may not have been the reason for the unusual round building at Epidauros south of the temple, the *tholos*; only three or four other such round buildings are known in antiquity. Interestingly, one of those is also at an Asklepios shrine, in Asia Minor (see n. 20). The *tholos* was supported on foundations in six concentric rings, made from volcanic tufa. (The suggestion that sacred snakes would have been kept there ignores reptiles' need for periodic exposure to light to regulate their body temperature). The floor, which had an elegant compass-drawn pattern, had a hole in it. Was the hole for sacrificial offerings to the hero Asklepios? The Asklepieion at Athens did not have a circular building but did have a circular pit, still visible.

¹⁶ IG II2 1252 and 1253. Sophocles was the author of the majestic tragedy *Oedipus the King,* which deals extensively with a great plague.

[17] Strangely kept locked; who knows why? Orthodox Christian Greece remains a conservative country. Myriad plaster forms of breasts along with genitalia of both genders accompany other forms of feet, hands, arms, and eyes.

[18] Miller, *Dreams in Late Antiquity,* 106.

[19] Edelstein and Edelstein, *Asclepius* I, T. 318: 163–164, attested as well by Clement of Alexandria, *Stromateis* 5.1.13, *Asclepius* I, T. 336: 177–78.

[20] The Asklepieion in the metropolis of Pergamon in Asia Minor, modern Turkey, was founded from Epidauros in the fourth century B.C.E.. In other words, it was a mission church that soon outstripped its mother church, becoming the leading cult center of Asklepios. It featured a mysterious round building that has the same shape as the *tholos* at Epidauros but that seemed to have had a very different function: this may have been, in fact, the two-story *abaton.* It has rock-cut channels running through its floors for carrying water.

[21] Aelius Aristides, *The Sacred Tales* 2: 32–33, trans. C. A. Behr, *Aelius Aristides and the Sacred Tales*, 230.

[22] Ibid. 1: 69–72, *Aelius Aristides,* 220–221.

[23] Ibid. 3: 15, *Aelius Aristides,* 244.

[24] Ibid. 2: 29–31, *Aelius Aristides,* 229.

[25] Carl Alfred Meier, *Ancient Incubation and Modern Psychotherapy*, trans. Monica Curtis (Evanston, IL: Northwestern University Press, 1967), 216.

[26] Edelstein and Edelstein, *Asclepius* I, T. 423: 221–237.

[27] Ibid., 322: 164.

[28] Meier, *Ancient Incubation and Modern Psychotherapy,* 66.

[29] A version of the preceding discussion of possession appeared in my article, "'A Great And Strange Correction': Intentionality, Locality, And Epiphany in the Category of Dream Incubation," *History Of Religions* 43: 3 (2004): 194 –223.

[30] Behr, *Aelius Aristides and the Sacred Tales,* 36, n. 64. IG IV2 1, nos. 121–122 (Edelstein and Edelstein, *Asclepius* I, T 423).

[31] Carl Alfred Meier, "The Dream in Ancient Greece and its Use in Temple Cures (Incubation)," in *The Dream and Human Societies,* ed. G. E. von Grunebaum and Roger Caillois (Berkeley: Univ. Cal. Press, 1966): 317.

[32] Michael Kearney, *A Place of Healing: Working with Suffering in Living and Dying* (Oxford University Press, 2000).

[33] Kelly Bulkeley and Patricia Bulkeley, *Dreaming Beyond Death: A Guide to Pre-Death Dreams and Visions* (Boston: Beacon Press, 2005).

[34] Ibid., 63 and n. 34.

[35] Edelstein and Edelstein, *Asclepius* I, T. 419: 211–212.

[36] Behr, *Aelius Aristides and the Sacred Tales,* 37 and nn. 68 and 69.

[37] Eldelstein and Edelstein, *Asclepius* II, 163.

[38] Ibid., 172.

[39] E. R. Dodds, *The Greeks and the Irrational* (Berkeley: University of California Press, [1951], 1968), 103.

[40] Edelsteins, *Asclepius* II, 162.

[41] E.g., T. J. Kaptchuk, "Powerful Placebo: The Dark Side of the Randomized Controlled Trial," *Lancet* 351 (1998): 1722–5; F. G. Miller and T. J. Kaptchuk, "The Power of Context: Reconceptualizing the Placebo Effect," *Journal of the Royal Society of Medicine* 101 (2008): 222–225.

[42] E.g., Tor D. Wager, "The Neural Bases of Placebo Effects in Pain," *Current Directions in Psychological Science* 14: 4 (2005): 175–179, etc.

[43] E.g., E. M. Sternberg and J. I. Webster, "Neural Immune Interactions in Health and Disease," in *Fundamental Immunology,* 5th ed., ed. W. E. Paul (Philadelphia: Lippincott Williams & Wilkins, 2003): 1021–1042; A. Deak and E. M. Sternberg, "Brain-immune Interactions and Disease Susceptibility," *Molecular Psychiatry* 2005: 1–12.

[44] Miller, *Dreams in Late Antiquity,* 115–116.

[45] Talal Asad, *Genealogies of Religion: Discipline and Reasons of Power in Christianity and Islam* (Baltimore and London: Johns Hopkins Univ. Press, 1993), esp. 75–77 on Marcel Mauss.

[46] Groopman, *How Doctors Think,* 18. Emphasis mine.

[47] Arthur Kleinman, *The Illness Narratives: Suffering, Healing, and the Human Condition* (New York : Basic Books, 1988).

2

Healing the Soul in a Culture of Fear

M I C H A E L   K E A R N E Y ,   M . D .

A lot of sick people go to our hospitals, and nowhere else, in their search for cure and for healing. Each night, each patient in the hospital dreams. And in the morning their dreams are ignored or, if noticed at all, are usually seen as a troublesome or irrelevant side effect of medication, a useless symptom to be further medicated. It does not have to be like this.

James was just recently transferred back to the floor. He had been admitted to hospital a week previously with a heart attack. While still in the critical care unit, this frail, seventy-seven-year-old man began to complain of problems with swallowing. Investigations showed this to be due to a large, inoperable carcinoma of the esophagus. As a member of the hospital's palliative care team, I was now visiting James to see what suggestions we might have to improve his comfort and to offer emotional support to him and his family.

James was so breathless from his resolving chest infection on top of his chronic pulmonary disease that he was unable to finish his sentences. He appeared frightened and anxious and when asked what he understood of his illness, he made it clear that he did not know and did not want to know: "I had a heart attack. As soon as this chest infection clears, I am going to go home. You can help me with that."

We left the ward having made some recommendations of medication that could help his shortness of breath and help him get some sleep at night. It was the weekend, and we did not get to revisit James until the following Monday afternoon. On arriving on the ward, I asked the charge nurse how James was doing. He replied that James had initially done a little better after our visit and after starting on the new meds but that the previous night he had awakened very distressed with a nightmare, calling out for his family, and that it had taken the night nurse a long time to persuade him to accept some Valium, which did eventually get him back to sleep.

I pulled a chair over and reached out a hand. Touching his arm I called James' name, saying, "Hi, James. It's Dr. Kearney . . . We met last Friday. I am sorry to hear you had a distressing nightmare last night." James, who until then had been lying on his side facing away from me with his eyes closed, slowly opened his eyes. He began to uncurl himself and ever so slowly sat up in his bed and turned to face me. "That was not a nightmare," he replied. "That was the most extraordinary dream I have had in my life." I was struck by the calm clarity in his voice. I replied, "Wow! I would love to hear about it if you would like to tell me."

"Last night I was sad as I went to sleep," he began. "A man in our ward had died earlier in the evening. It got me thinking about some of my own family who have passed on this past year. It seemed like I had just got off to sleep when I felt someone put their hand on my arm, just like you did a minute ago. When I looked up there was this man, about my age, dressed in a black suit. He wore glasses, and he told me his name was Professor John Kelly Reeves. He said he did not have long to live and that there was something he wanted to show me before he died.

He took me to New Grange [a Neolithic burial chamber over four thousand years old]. *He asked me to go inside, to walk down the underground tunnel to the central chamber. He told me to put my back to the back wall of the tomb* [this is the precise spot that is illuminated just once a year at Midwinter Solstice]. *Then he told me to take thirty steps down the tunnel that brought me outside. It was dark. He asked me to take seven steps to the left, then another seven steps. Then he handed me a shovel and asked me to start digging. Pretty soon I hit rocks, and I began to see the outline of circular houses, then the straight lines of a road. I began to realize that under New Grange was a city—a pre-ancient city! I felt like I'd struck gold! I wanted to tell my family all about it!"*

I listened in awe, in wonder at the dream, for sure, but even more so at the incredible change I was witnessing in James himself. It was hard to recognize this man who spoke full sentences with a quiet authority, whose dark, hollowed eyes appeared filled with light, as the same frightened man I had met just days before.

James was clearly proud of his dream. He loved to talk about it and did so on every occasion we met over the following two weeks. On what was to turn out to be the day before he died, I visited James once again. It was clear that his condition had weakened considerably and that, unfortunately, he would not going to be able to make it home again. While he had never spoken openly about his deteriorating condition, he made arrangements to finish making his will. Once again he launched into talking about his dream. Looking straight ahead he said, "You know . . . when that professor said that he did not have long to live, maybe he meant that I did not have long to live. In any case, it does not really matter now. Since I had the dream, I'm not frightened anymore." James died peacefully the following day, his wife and sons at his bedside.

What happened here is what happened every night at Epidauros, at Pergamun, at Lissos: James had incubated a healing dream. While the dream did not cure his cancer, it did dissolve his fear and allow him to experience a deeper sense of what Mount calls "healing connections"[1] that carried him peacefully through his final days. What enabled this to happen? Good care lessened his fear and helped to create a secure-enough space in which his innate potential towards integration, inclusiveness, and wholeness could manifest. He had experienced an epiphany of healing.

In this article I propose that wholeness is already there; that it is fear that separates and that our task as healers is to remember what already is. If this is correct and wholeness and interconnectedness are *a priori*, then sickness, disease, and illness are what happen when we become alienated from this reality. Within this understanding, healing is a reconnecting with our native state. However simple this may sound, we would be naïve to think that healing is necessarily an easy matter. It may be or it may not be, depending on a number of variables, including how great an individual's fear is and the type and quality of care that person receives. The question of healing comes into stark relief in the microcosm of end-of-life care. Here we must begin by coming to a deeper understanding of the dynamics of the dying ego.

TERROR MANAGEMENT THEORY

Terror Management Theory (TMT) evolved from a process of trying to understand why social and cultural minorities are persecuted. For over thirty years Solomon, Greenberg, and Pyszczynski have been field-testing their hypothesis, which draws on the pioneering work of Pulitzer Award-winning author Ernest Becker and his book, *The Denial of Death*.[2] Their research is well-summarized in the book, *In the Wake of 911: The Psychology of Terror*[3] and the award-winning documentary movie *Flight from Death*.[4]

In essence, TMT postulates that because awareness of death is intolerable to humans, it is repressed. Additionally, to protect against this, humans have constructed culture. To have a meaningful place in this culture is to be part of something "bigger" that was there before and will be there after a human lifetime; in other words, it is a way of experiencing symbolic immortality, which buffers that individual from terror of annihilation. There is, therefore, a powerful drive to maintain the culture we are part of because it is protecting us from our deepest fears. When something comes along that threatens that culture, we react in a variety of ways designed to defend our culture (the "dominant culture" in TMT), referred to as "terror management processes." These involve (1) distancing ourselves from the threat (the "minority culture" in TMT); (2) attempting to disarm the threat by finding ways of assimilating small portions of it into the culture; and (3) if the first two methods fail, acting to eliminate the threat. TMT research also shows that reminders of mortality ("mortality salience" in TMT) trigger these same terror management processes. In other words, reminders of our mortality make us reactionary and defensive around our culture and its values because something in us senses that life as we know it depends on this.

In terms of the individual Western psyche, the dominant cultural values are those of rational and concrete thinking. Mortality salience terrifies the ego, which now becomes the organizing principle of the psyche. It retreats to the safety of the familiar ("dominant culture") in the form of rationalism, materialism, and literal thinking and away from the unfamiliar ("minority culture") in the form of body, depth, complexity, intuition, and direct experience. This in turn leads to dissociation and alienation. Perhaps the ego recognizes in the unfamiliar darkness of the unconscious a microcosm of the great unknown, the ultimate darkness: death. As Jung puts it: *"The dread and resistance which every natural human being experiences when it comes to delving too deeply into himself is, at bottom, the fear of the journey into Hades."*[5] While distancing from psychological depth may have short-term beneficial effects by giving the terrified ego a sense of control, these are, at best, short-lived. What is more, this results in an ego that is disconnected from the healing potential of the deep psyche, leading to an experience of alienation, isolation, and meaninglessness: "soul pain."[6]

The possibility that terror management processes are also active at a collective level within Western health care would help to explain the dehumanizing excesses of technological medicine as the defensive activities of terrified human egos make mortality salient by constant proximity to disease and death. It also explains the complete dominance of the medical model within health care since this closely reflects dominant cultural values. This might also help us to understand why a splitting occurs between the medical model and therapeutic approaches such as dream work that embody the values of the minority culture: those of the deep psyche. At best such approaches are denigrated as "soft" (i.e., tolerated within the system but, by implication, not really that important or relevant in the real world of "hard data"); at worst they are trashed as useless or even dangerous.

CARE OF THE DYING EGO

So how can we care for the dying ego? Little is possible unless we begin with a compassionate understanding of what is happening here and realize that we are dealing with an ego that is desperately hanging, like some scared animal, to the ceiling of consciousness, disconnected from the potentially healing depths of psyche. Henry Miller lyrically describes the challenge now facing the ego in the following passage:

> At Epidauros, in the stillness, in the great peace that came over me, I heard the heart of the world beat. I know what the cure is: it is to give up, to relinquish, to surrender, so that our little hearts may beat in unison with the great heart of the world.[7]

To find healing, in other words, the ego has to let go.

There are two possibilities at this point. The first, and perhaps the more common, is that the ego holds on for all it is worth. And it continues to do so until the floodwaters of impending doom rise so high as to overwhelm its grip. This first way is the way of drowning ego. The tragedy here is twofold. First, it may involve additional unnecessary suffering for that individual and those close to him or her. Second, it may not allow that individual to realize the potential of such a time in his or her life for growth and healing. There is another way. This way involves the choice to let go. It is the way of descent. To paraphrase Jung, it is the way of diving rather than drowning. Phil Simmons, in an address at Harvard Medical School shortly before his death from amyotrophic lateral sclerosis, put it this way:

> At its deepest level life is not a problem but a mystery. The distinction is fundamental: problems are solved, mysteries are not. At one time or another, each of us confronts an experience so powerful, bewildering, joyous, or terrifying, that all our efforts to see it as a problem are futile. Each of reaches the end of reason's rope. And when we do, we can either grip harder and get nowhere, or we can let go, and fall. For what does mystery ask of us? Only that we be in its presence, that we fully, consciously, hand ourselves over. That is all, and that is everything.[8]

What can we do as caregivers to facilitate our patients' letting go in this way? The first step in this process is hinted at by Cicely Saunders, founder of the modern hospice movement, when she draws a distinction between *safety* and *security:*

> The real presence of another person is a place of security. I recall remarking to two psychiatrists that when patients are in a climate of safety they will come to realize what is happening in their own way and not be afraid. One said: "How can you speak of a climate of safety when death is the most unsafe thing that can happen?" To which the other replied: "I think you are using the wrong word. I think it should be "security." A child separated from his mother may be quite safe—but he feels very insecure. A child in his mother's arms during an air raid may be very unsafe indeed—but he feels quite secure. We have to give all patients that feeling of security in which they can begin, when they are ready, to face unsafety.[9]

To facilitate a letting go to depth, in other words, we must begin by creating a secure-enough container for the terrified ego. While it may be too big a step for the terrified ego to let go directly to the unknown, it may be possible for the ego to choose to let go to the secure-enough container of care.

THE CONTAINER OF CARE

The relationship that is formed between caregiver and patient is the therapeutic container in which healing occurs; it is a channel for empathy, compassion, and reassurance; it is the secure space in which the ego may begin to loosen its grip. There are three dynamic components of the container of care. These are: what we do; how we do what we do; and who we are as caregivers.

What We Do

Our knowledge and skills as caregivers determine our clinical effectiveness. Through the curative and palliative interventions we perform for our patients, through the psychosocial interventions we offer them and their families, and through competently planning and organizing their care, we lessen fear, offer comfort, and build trust. By our expertly treating problems, appropriate and effective therapeutic interventions help to create the preconditions that facilitate letting go.

How We Do What We Do

Our identity as healers is primarily shaped by our attitudes, perception, and quality of care we offer than by a particular knowledge base and skill set. As Saunders observes, "The way care is given can reach the most hidden places and give space for unexpected development."[10] Healing is about doing what we are already doing for our patients with a new attitude, one that understands the deeper narrative of what is unfolding rather than necessarily doing new or different things. The way care is given can reassure the insecure ego.

Who We Are as Persons

Psychiatrist Michael Balint talks about the "doctor [caregiver] as drug."[11] He suggests that who we caregivers are as persons (as opposed to our professional persona) is the most potent medicine we give our patients. Continuing with this metaphor, he suggests that we know far less about this drug—in terms of how it works, its interactions, and side effects—than we do about most any other medication in our pharmacopoeia. Who we are as persons determines both the quality of our relationships and the quality of the care we offer our patients.

Dying Whole

Jungian analyst Albert Kreinheder chronicles his experience of living and dying with chronic illness in his beautiful book, *Body and Soul: The Other Side of Illness.*[12] He writes:

> There is a way to die. It doesn't matter when you die so much as how you die. Not by what means but whether or not you are in one piece, psychologically speaking. I remember frequently those words of Kieffer: "The object of healing is not to stay alive. The object of healing is to become more whole. Death is the final healing."[13]

In the final pages of the book Kreinheder reminds us of the other side of the healing story; that it's not all about the ego. The soul has its own narrative that is unfolding independently of the ego's chatter as we live with illness and as we approach death. There is care of the frightened and dying ego, and there is ongoing care of the emerging soul. Kreinheder writes:

> Our little time within this body is soon over, but life in its larger sense goes on. The knowledge of our rapidly approaching death makes us more aware of that other realm where dwell the saints and archetypes. When we are no longer afraid of death, we are also unafraid of the archetypes, and their power comes marching into our lives.[14]

In addition to caring for the dying ego in all the ways we have been discussing, Kreinheder encourages us to spend time with soul:

> The more we are with soul, the less identified we are with the ego. We know our center to be a larger stream of life transcending ego and going on beyond our death. The soul is somehow in union with this larger being. And as I align myself more with soul and less with ego, the soul's story becomes my story. Then I cannot grieve unduly for the ego. It is like a candle that has had its hour and now must flicker and go out.[15]

Surely this is not just a prescription for dying. It is a prescription for healing. And it is encouragement to embrace more deeply our "one wild and precious life."[16]

NOTES

[1] B. Mount, "Healing Connections: On Moving from Suffering to a Sense of Well-Being," *Journal of Pain and Symptom Management* 33, no. 4 (April 2007): 372–388.

[2] E. Becker, *The Denial of Death* (New York: Free Press Paperbacks, 1992).

[3] S. Solomon, J. Greenberg, and T. Pyszczynski, *In the Wake of 9/11: The Psychology of Terror* (Washington, DC: American Psychological Association, 2003).

[4] P. Shen, and G. Bennick, *Flight From Death: The Quest for Immortality,* DVD, (Transcendental Media, 2005).

[5] C. G. Jung, *Psychology and Alchemy,* trans. R. F. C. Hull, vol. 12 of *The Collected Works of C. G.* Jung (Princeton, NJ: Princeton Univ. Press, 1953), 439.

✓ [6] M. Kearney, *Mortally Wounded: Stories of Soul Pain, Death and Healing* (New Orleans: Spring Journal Books, 2007).

[7] H. Miller, *The Colossus of Maroussi* (New York: New Directions, 1941), 79.

[8] P. Simmons (address, Harvard Medical School, Cambridge, MA, March 20, 2001).

[9] C. Saunders, *The Management of Terminal Disease* (London: Edward Arnold, 1976), 6.

[10] C. Saunders, "Foreword," in *Mortally Wounded: Stories of Soul Pain, Death and Healing.*

[11] M. Balint, *The Doctor, His Patient and the Illness* (Edinburgh: Churchill Livingstone, 2000).

✓ [12] A. Kreinheder, *Body and Soul: The Other Side of Illness* (Toronto: Inner City Books, 1991).

[13] Ibid., 108.

[14] Ibid.

[15] Ibid., 109.

[16] M. Oliver, "The Summer Day," in *New and Selected Poems* (Boston, MA: Beacon Press, 1992).

Water Spirits, Multiple Sclerosis, and Poisoned of a God

MICHAEL ORTIZ HILL

Sacred illness is first and foremost *poesis*. Flesh rendered poem, praise song, lament. And so I begin and end this essay with poetry.

This I wrote after my last multiple sclerosis exacerbation. Losing my legs, losing my mind with steroid therapy. Recovering my legs with steroid therapy and, weaned from decadron, recovering a portion of my mind. In this, Spirit prepared me in its fierce and generous way to accompany a few Vietnam vets and fellow travelers like myself to Vietnam with Dr. Ed Tick for healing and reconciliation.

Amalgam: Hope/Hopelessness

Beginning of summer
Darkness revealed by harshness of light
Surprised by fright of old friend death
Lust for old enemy
the longing for the last breath
Now equinox double ought six
Hope tempered by hopelessness
Hopelessness tempered by possibility of hope
Tranquil heart of mandala
Multiple sclerosis
And soon I will be with the beggars of Saigon

Sacred illness is firstly *poesis*: to be conceived in the body of metaphor, gestate there, birthed perhaps in this life or through death. Among my people in Africa, the Shona and the Ndebele (Zulu) of Zimbabwe, sacred illness comes of God and returns to God in this life or through the end of it. Healing can mean either. The essential thing is to listen to the spirit that afflicts, yield to its wisdom, be undone as one will be undone, be stripped and stripped again to what is most elemental and true, most true and most uncertain.

I will write here of three sacred afflictions: water spirit disease, multiple sclerosis, and the spirit of etiology—poisoned with the God Mercury, Mercurius, the one the Yoruba call Eshu Elegba.

These three are interrelated—in fact, continuous with one another.

WATER SPIRIT ILLNESS

In the early 1990s I began gathering racial dreams: white people's dreams about black people, the dreams of blacks about whites. I wanted to honor the dreams of black Americans by looking at them through the wisdom traditions of Mother Africa.

As I went further into my studies of the African origins of black America it became clear that whites were being dreamt within the same field of imagery that western Bantu people had understood as "whiteness" since the Portuguese friars turned up in the kingdom of the Kongo in the fifteenth century.

In *The Village of the Water Spirits: The Dreams of African-Americans*,[1] I look to the tribal strata beneath the African diaspora in America and particularly the seminal water spirit tradition. It was Melville Herskovits in 1941 who was the first to note that the primary ritual of black Baptist culture in America, full immersion baptism, was African in origin. The "intransigence of the priests of the river cult," wrote Herskovits, "was so marked that more than any other group of holy men, they were sold into slavery to rid the conquerors of troublesome leaders."[2]

The *ngoma* of the water spirits was once the sacred way of royalty and persists today in healing ceremonials and peacemaking. Anthropologists call the way of the water spirits a cult of affliction. "The stitch of pain leads to the village of the ancestors," says the Bakongo proverb. The understanding is that the *midzimu*—the invisibles—call one to being a *nganga* (healer) through water spirit illness.

After years of preparation, I found myself in the house of Mandaza Kandemwa in Bulawayo, Zimbabwe.

(Who was this white stranger who had traveled thousands of miles knowing himself to be called to the way of water?)

Who, indeed. It's been years now of the piercing initiations through sacred illness and only now am I beginning to understand the strange ways of the boy I was. The boy would say simply, "I was called." True enough, but when I saw Africa inherent in the nightly dreams of black Americans I knew I had been called to Africa to bring back the gift of a tribal dreamteller understanding of these dreams.

Mandaza seemed to recognize me on our first meeting. "You are a typical water spirit person," he said. All the symptoms: vivid dreams and waking visions, afflicted with an empathy that incapacitates, swings of emotion, stomach problems, a life rich in tragedy.

The only cure for water spirit disease is initiation as a healer and ritual practitioner into the *ngoma* of the water spirits. As this is a peace-making tradition, one begins by making peace with the spirit that afflicts. Only then can the water spirits be allies in the activity of healing—one's own healing through perpetuity of initiation, and the healing of others.

MULTIPLE SCLEROSIS

Forgive that I quote at length the book I wrote with my wife Deena Metzger, *Sacred Illness, Sacred Medicine*.[3]

"My apprenticeship with multiple sclerosis began very slowly, retrospect being the only angle from which one might even see its beginnings. I was in Africa in 1996 with my wife introducing her to the Bantu people who had initiated and received me as a medicine man. We were in the stony waterlands of Mashvingo, southern Zimbabwe. Deena was initiating Mandaza into the mysteries of the Hebrew letters, when I noted a garden variety of white male arrogance rising up in me. After all, I was 'the expert,' much a part of the tribal world and quite well read on Bantu anthropology. How much I wanted to interfere, be master of ceremonies. So I pulled away to a small pool of water to curl up in and prayed in the traditional way of the *ngoma* of the water spirits. I yielded to the field of spirits that were carrying the poetry of the moment quite without my advice. It was then the snail parasite schistosoma slid through the skin and apparently laid eggs in the lattice of my nervous system.

"That night a fever, strange but transient; two weeks later, numb from the waist down. And so I walked eight years with this numbness. Eighty percent of peripheral neuropathies are undiagnosable, I was told. With reluctance, accustomed to a young man's oblivious vigor, I settled into the constant reminder of the frailty of the flesh.

"All this started changing when I lost the full use of my legs. It was then that my apprenticeship with the sacred illness, soon to be named multiple sclerosis, truly began. How fortunate I am that MS insinuated itself into my body at a moment of surrender, and has kept such perfect faith with the teaching of surrender, and surrender, and yet again, surrender. And then there are the gifts that come in the wake of surrender.

"Surrender? What do I mean by surrender? Anagarika Sujata says that there is dishonesty in any mind that insists reality occur in a specific way. MS says that healing requires a strange alliance with what I am facing, and so the way of surrender has demanded an uncompromising honesty. Not a passive acceptance, but a very active meeting.

"My first serious rendezvous with the spirit of the illness was last August 2005, when I walked to the cave on the Big Sur coast where I'd been blessed to spend two years during my twenties and thirties in solitude and meditation. It took me ten hours to walk what had been a one-hour hike. In my two weeks alone I surrendered my legs, not knowing if they'd return or even if I'd be able to make my way out of the ravine. Later I surrendered my life. Undiagnosed as yet, I didn't know if that time had come. Finally, there was surrendering the fetish of certainty, knowing that God is the one who shapes what is before me. Such has been my spiritual practice during this time, and through it I have begun to taste freedom.

"Occasionally!

"Surrendering my legs, perplexed that I would be asked to do so, but with whom do I argue? Surrendering my life was a different matter, that truculent fantasy that my life and my death are possessions of mine, body be damned. Deena is twenty years my senior, and there have been many years of renewing the vow that I'd see her to the other side—a betrayal of her and God's betrayal of both of us should our lot be otherwise. But yes, the tearful moment five minutes before the New Year's kiss, insisting that she continue should I go first.

"The third lesson from the illness was surrendering the fetish of certainty. A few months ago I was delivered vividly between worlds. I was between lives, one life dead and gone and the next unborn, that place the Tibetans call bardo. Flailing in rage, indulging in an orgiastic fit of self-pity, and Deena, bless her, said, 'You have to let go of how you think and talk about these things.' The space of the bardo echoed with the 'let go, let go, let go' as if to harangue. I knew that spiritually I seem to be called to let go of most everything, or perhaps merely any shard of certainty.

"Ah, the Fool card of the Tarot! My father gave me my first Tarot deck before he died, and I've long used it to understand my fate. Did I not see the Fool as a photograph of my soul, satchel at the end of a stick stepping over a cliff, dog nipping at my heels? Did I not always yearn to dance at the edge of the abyss? And yet, quite denying now years of my public and private rhetoric that could well be the fiction of having a self, I'm seduced by the fetish of certainty—that fetish that I've always scoffed at with contempt. Affectionate though he was towards the young man's flamboyance, now he places the older man's meditation cushion at the edge of the uncertainty that has become his life and says, 'Sit still.'

"How little I've understood the Fool. A little psychosis, a bit of entertainment, half-time in the rites of surrender. I'm left with the question, stripped bare—what is the authentic and ensouled truth of the story I am in?"

Such was my first rendezvous, the beginning of making an alliance with multiple sclerosis. A year later I was cast to sea in what Mandaza would call "proper initiation."

Exacerbation.

Thank God my *ngoma* initiation had taught me a little about befriending a spirit.

The rite of descent was relentless—dis-membering who I thought I was and re-membering slow and thorough. In *Meeting Sacred Illness*[4] I try to give words to it:

"And this initiation into sacred illness? How does one speak of the illness that undoes one even as it heals? How does one tell the story about the undoing of one's story? Who is the self that bears witness to the undoing of the self? Does one contrive a self to tell the story? And who is this contrived self? Is he at all an honorable fellow? A trustworthy witness?

"All lies in retrospect and all retrospect lies. The land of memory is terra incognita but what of the land of the disintegration of the memories that I knew as terra firma? The place of memory is always contested ground, isn't it? What is true? And what a tissue of lies rendered believable?

"In this lonely place do I sing the body electric, the gimpy walk, the curious torque of mind? Do I sing through the invisible wound that so shapes me, the lesions in my brain stem, frontal lobe, corpus collosum, trailing down the core of my spine through throat and heart chakra? This wound some call multiple sclerosis I call the Guest. MS is an autoimmune disease. The self attacking the self. For that reason I cannot call the Guest an enemy. The deep questions are how to be hospitable to one so fierce in his wisdom.

"Dare I encourage the Guest to sing?

"Dare I not?"

The Guest's song is nigredo. Putrefaction. Decomposition. The vertigo of the mirror of oneself facing a thousand mirrors: three decades of patients covered in shit and now myself beshitted. People I have cared for unable to string together a coherent sentence and now I was unable. Staggering. Falling. Getting up and falling again. Eyes failing. The dissolution of a couple of months of sleeplessness and the spurious omnipotence of decadron psychosis.

I went to the forest for a few weeks alone to make sense of it. There I read a transcript of Deena's keynote address at the American Holistic Medical Association conference called "The Soul of Medicine."

"Michael sometimes speaks of the spirit of MS," said Deena. "He means that he, as patient and healer, is apprenticing to the disease and what it reveals about the needs and nature of the body and the body politic. MS is an inflammatory autoimmune disease of the central nervous system wherein damaged nerve fibers are unable to fully or reliably transmit communication signals to the rest of the body. It is a disease on the rise in a society, a world, that is enraged, violent, and militant ... . We think Michael succumbed to MS because we must learn to heal our inflamed hearts and souls and he has the capacity to address this. Don't give yourself to being healed until you know the story of the disease," says Deena.

In solitude I wrote my response:

"I couldn't quite understand these words when she spoke them. Perhaps this is the way with disease. It inheres so much in your character that you are the last to see it—until you fall apart. Decadron!

The great anti-inflammatory! What, me inflamed? Inflammatory? On fire? Setting fires? Playing with fire? Sweet, pacifist, Buddhist hippie me? And yet my life tells the story of an inflamed sense of self, fire forever seeking more fire, forever the nostalgia for Vietnam, knowing it only in my nightmares. Hearth and home for me has been mostly the stoking of hearth. I was most myself in the flames."[5]

I groaned when Deena called decadron "my sacred medicine," but have come to call her *ambuya* (Shona for grandmother) and to ritually engage her in those rare, bitter seasons when I've had to partake. Her dark blessing is that she shows shadow—sometimes flagrantly, publicly. Visibly undeniable, and by virtue of that softening to hospitality that the Guest might be at ease.

EPISTEMOLOGICAL INTERLUDE

There is a path between one medical way and another, a path I learned to walk those years I practiced as a registered nurse and *nganga* at UCLA Medical Center. Of such a path the Yoruba have a parable, about Eshu Elegba.

They say there were two friends who were initiated together among the boys and, as men, tilled the soil together in adjacent fields. They were inseparable, they thought, kin beyond the blood of it and they often praised such a friendship.

Eshu decided to play a trick. Painting one side of his face black and the other white he sauntered down the path between the fields as each friend hoed their respective plots.

"Who was that strange white man?" one asked across the path.

"White man? White man? That man was coal black. That was no white man."

"What, you crazy? I know a white man when I see a white man."

It went like this, got hotter and hotter until the two were wrestling in the mud.

Eshu Elegba loves to undo us in our certainties because in our certainties we are most blind. In our certainties we are deaf to the sacred nature of what afflicts, deaf to the profound intelligence of what ails us.

His persistent and sometimes cutting wisdom reveals what is eclipsed by certainty.

THE SPIRIT OF ETIOLOGY

Who is Eshu Elegba?

Several years before I was initiated into the *ngoma* of the water spirits, I was "in the ashes" of race relations in Los Angeles. Just two months after the Rodney King riots/uprising I was taken by Eshu Elegba, the Yoruba spirit of the crossroad. He or I took the form of a "mobius strip." For a couple of hours I writhed alone on the living room carpet—he becoming I; then I, he. I'd sob over the hell of race and he'd taunt, "Whassup with the blues song white boy?" and then, flipside, undone with laughter, "What you laughing about now?"

Back and forth, my first undoing by an African spirit. The Lord of the roads and keeper of the doorway, he carried me into the mysteries of the many faces of God, the *orisha*.

I've named a dozen common motifs between Eshu and Hermes/ Mercury. (It seems likely that by way of Egyptian Tehuti/Thoth this spirit found his way across the Sahara and the Sahel to west Africa.) There was a thud of the inevitable when I tested extremely high for mercury. I had a complex ritual relationship with Eshu/Mercury, within which I received the allopathic etiology for multiple sclerosis. I was thickly mercurial, toxic via dental amalgams since childhood and to a measure before birth. Mercury torques/shapes the nervous system in the fetus. I was conceived in iatrogenesis and as far as I can tell birthed as his Siamese twin.

European Catholicism assimilated Hermes as St. Michael the Archangel. Likewise in Haiti Eshu became St. Michael.

Thus my flesh has a certain intimacy with the god, but the fleet-footed god entangled, imprisoned in my body, enraged. The god made poison.

That blasphemy. That arrogance.

The Yoruba consider Eshu Elegba the spirit of the individual self— its idiosyncrasies, passions, flaws. The way it dances the sacred. This is also true of the alchemical Mercurius who Jung saw as the archetype of one's individual nature.

To be poisoned by the mercurial leads to self-devouring breakdown, having an almost allergic reaction to one's peculiar familiar self. Most curious mania: Mercury and I inseparable, maddening one another. Pathophysiologically the portrait is autoimmune. In my case— multiple sclerosis.

Alchemically the *poesis* of mercury toxicity renders the body an alembic. There is again the nigredo of breakdown: all piss and shit. And then there is separation—chelation—ultimately leaving the god's quintessence, for his residue remains. One cannot completely expunge the god. Mercury remains as ally.

Something began shifting when I started separating mercury from my central nervous system—that holy of holies. A mercy for the god himself arose, that he might be exorcised of me, that he might be set free from the dank prison that I am.

Thus separation—the strange, sometimes hallucinatory absorption of "me and my demon"—untangles to the obvious. The refining of Mercury to quintessence in the alembic of my life delivers me to solidarity with a poisoned world, a solidarity with we citizens of the food chain who so like eating one another.

In the environment mercury finds itself in the sludge of streams and bacteria methylates it—converts it to its most toxic form.

Likewise, in the eco-niche of a person's mouth the oral bacteria methylates the mercury of dental amalgams. Amalgams are 60% mercury.

I've come to feel affectionate towards the "little ones" that have so composed my life: schistosoma entering at the ritual moment of surrender, and the tireless labor of millions of generations of bacteria delivering mercury to the pit of my karma. They are most certainly water spirits. It seems that the bacteria that made me mercurial softened my nervous system so that schistosoma could erode and inflame the myelin sheaths for the ritual descent into multiple sclerosis.

Schistosoma – water spirit illness – multiple sclerosis – bacteria and methylated mercury poisoning is a single syndrome, capacious enough to accommodate the Bantu and the allopathic. From the Bantu point of view the path is clear. The *ngoma* of the water spirits is a healing and peacemaking tradition. To make peace is to heal. To heal is to make peace. Make an alliance with that which would kill and let that alliance work through you that you might, perhaps, practice as a healer.

It is the essence of anthropomorphic narcissism to imagine my body is the locus of poisoning. I cannot forget to sing gratitude to the spirit that afflicts, for it is that spirit which even now is initiating. Such is the craft of the schistosoma and bacteria that I've been cracked open to the vulnerability of this dear planet.

I spent a few months alone inviting my fifth decade with meditation and ritual on the Big Sur coast. Every morning I'd gather seaweed, sea snails, chitons, gooseneck barnacles. I'd dry them on a river rock and mix them with my evening ramen. After offering a tablespoon to the deer mice I'd glut on my nightly mercury.

My beloved California is mercurial. Abandoned mercury mines upstream in the Los Padres National Forest and further to the east, the Sierras.

In the eighteenth century those rude alchemists, the "forty-niners," flooded the food chain with mercury used to process gold. And in the early nineteenth century mercury amalgams were first placed in people's mouths.

In 1868 Jean-Martin Charcot first named multiple sclerosis as a clinical phenomenon.

It is said that a third of the airborne mercury in the San Francisco Bay is from cremation. Vaporized amalgams of the teeth of corpses.

The alembic again is this body, but most certainly also this fragile world. Of alchemical Mercury Robbie Bosnak writes, "From this dark, untrustworthy, poisonous and crafty being, the alchemist had to make the elixir, the remedy that consists of poison and of the poisoning that brings healing. They call it pharmacon, 'healing poison.'"[6]

There is a strangeness of being poisoned of a god and, within that god, living one's remembered life. Phillip K. Dick would be equal to the sinister, visionary truth of it. Mercury, as in "mad as a hatter," damn near toxic as plutonium placed in the mouths of children to leach into their minds its peculiar mind-altering ways.

I could never imagine how radically mind-altering systemic mercury was until I began to chelate it from my nervous system.

I began to notice that I live in a house and have done so since those years I was homeless. Quite simple, and absurdly startling. I wanted a little yogurt, walked across the kitchen, opened the fridge, and knew exactly where it was. I took it out and ate it.

Miraculous, no?

A couple of weeks later, eating cherries with my daughter Nicole, I inadvertently drop one; it bounces off the edge of the table and I snatch it in midair.

How marvelous. How utterly extraordinary!

I know this is the enlightenment of an imbecile, but the cascade of cognitive shifts continues to surprise. These elementary forms of cognition were much off the map for me. Locating things in space—the yogurt at the lower left side of the fridge, the cherry plump to the deft gaze, the quick hand. They are vivid to me, those studies linking mercury toxicity to autism. An autistic child can't imagine the reality of another human being. For myself, at the edge of the poison there was a solipsism that makes the world quite uncompelling, yet I had to forever improvise a relationship to it.

The first few weeks alone I struggled with the finding and refinement of the prayer of the leave-taking of mercury, his chalice a urinal.

I complete this essay from my cave among the redwood and madrone on the coast of California, where I'm alone for a couple of months inviting my sixth decade. There is much I cannot say, cannot even articulate to myself.

The first time I tried in earnest to call mercury from my central nervous system—cilantro extract, the medicine of choice—I was aggressive in my desire to be free and provoked a MS exacerbation. I've begun to learn slow and thorough the ritual craft of such a healing.

The first time I "emptied the chalice" I sang a Yoruba song to Eshu and talked to the crickets and tiny Argentinean black ants who then were my closest kin.

"This is poisonous. I am so sorry. Please stay away." Either they listened or they caught the scent of death.

In 1989, each American produced twenty-five tons of toxic waste—five hundred times more as per capita in 1973. I know what that meant as a nurse. A lot of children with cancer buried beneath a greedy economic putsch. A couple of grams of mercury poured from the fronds of my myelin sheaths is most certainly a pittance, but there is something unabashed and intimate to my frequent ritual offerings to my private waste dump.

Alchemically the process has been from the massa confusa of nigredo to separatio to the breaking of circulatio.

Perhaps an excruciating breaking of the heart, or maybe the heart of the world itself breaking. One cannot celebrate the offering of poison to a poisoned world.

Mercury has always been in circulation in me, but this in-breaking of circulatio declares the double alembic of my flesh, this planet.

In Buddhism the fiction of self is a trick played with mirrors, and before things began settling in my meditation practice the three stooges— "me, myself and I"—made almost operatic the passing of a little water.

Götterdämmerung!

But the ethical truth is non-dual. Short of passing water on another planet (Mercury?), there is nowhere to hide the alembic of my poisoned body nested into the alembic of a poisoned earth.

This life, brief as a flash of lightning, says the Diamond Sutra. (Ten years since I was alone like this, come and gone like a cup of coffee.)

The true and unplumbed healing takes place in the alembic set within the alembic of nature—nature and the fictitious "I" inseparable. My healing is inextricable from the healing of the earth.

This is the Bodhisattva vow—to practice this two-vessel alchemy until all beings a re liberated from the delusion of separateness. What remains of poison within me, may it transform to the nectar of compassion.

Everything began shifting a couple of weeks ago. The moon was darkening and I'd taken to "telling the rosary" of my MS lesions. I got up to empty the chalice after midnight and heard damned near audibly, "Your ancestors held slaves in Virginia and Georgia. Your contemporaries—the lot of you—are killing the earth." I felt a pinch in my brain stem, the primitive brain, medulla oblongata, and when it wouldn't let go I was frightened. I never physically felt the squeeze of a lesion, the pulse. My nurse self thought, "Am I provoking exacerbation? A stroke?"

This lesion bearing an ancestral wound, so utterly not of this life but also the lateral wound of living in an apocalyptic time and unable to lie about it.

I think of my black kin in America—those Hills and Halberts whom I've never broken bread with, and my black kin in Liberia, settled from the plantations before emancipation. Telling the rosary of my secret life, inadmissible.

When I was a boy I heard rumors of the *penetentes* in the mountains of Mora, not far from where we tilled corn. They flagellated themselves, some say crucified a man every Easter. It seems that an alter ego began his life then, devoted to the blood and the ecstasy. Decades of flagellating my central nervous system. I hum Leonard Cohen:

> "Forget about your perfect offering.
> There is a crack in everything
> That's how the light gets in."

The antics of the three stooges soon went silent. I stopped my Yoruba singing. Mercury became "have mercy," then just "mercy."

Mercury went through a change of character that I'm at a loss to describe. When we first came to be alone here the familiar horseplay between us would sometimes make me laugh when I was trying to meditate.

"What, you think this urinal is some great improvement to your precious nervous system: Chalice my ass! Let me out!"

Once he offered me some of that 181 proof rum he likes so much. I told him I'd rather drink sterno.

At first I was intrigued that his absence—or absenting—was such a vivid presence, but when Mercury became mercy he became the dust of a wandering thought, then random sensation.

As I was meditating a couple of days ago he and the Guest became figures in a limitless field, substantial as smoke, and it seemed quite untethered to my body. Also in the field were the phantoms of being healed or not being healed. Both plausible and implausible, but ultimately not worth investing much passion in.

Being taken by sacred illnesses is showing me that I hadn't a clue what the dimensions of healing are and maybe now I can live into it. The trail of water spirit disease, schistosoma, MS, and methylated mercury seems to have led me to this cave.

Mercury has become mercy and now—silence.

Cut for the Harvest

> For Ambuya Bwebwe and Mandaza Kandemwa

1

And I lie in bed
sleepless, raving, urinating on myself,
body slowly unravelling
how is it that Spirit plants medicine in the body
through illness?
multiple sclerosis
What is it through illness
utters wisdom
dares say the name
of the god that reweaves the world?

2

"Michael it is time you sing of how your body
has become medicine."
I trust now only what is small and true
the soft touch of the hand
the sudden light of the eyes
the impulse of the gut toward compassion
Love is the only medicine I know and I know it is not mine
passed swift from Lover to Beloved
weaving from hand to hand
the gift given
never owned
utterly ordinary and also, perhaps, a song
to those spirits knowing what healing is
healing as I most certainly do not

3

The Lover sometimes feeds on suffering
and of that the world is generous
I pray to which has made my life common and kind
that changes not water to wine
but wine to water
for refusing the common fate
we become thieves in the night
too dark to ourselves to see thief
or blinded by light
staggering unable to see blindness

4

First before the legs start giving way
before forgetting the English language
light sucked eyes dim can no longer discern
the mind of kin
wife beside me
twin ten thousand miles away
The body lost, stuttering

falling again and again

drooling, beshitting myself

Love is the only medicine

I have ever known

Have ever known

Love cut for the harvest

at last real in my own defeat

NOTES

[1] Michael Ortiz Hill, *The Village of the Water Spirits: The Dreams of African-Americans* (Spring Publications, 2006).

[2] Melville J. Herskovits, *The Myth of the Negro Past* (Boston: Beacon Press, 1941), 35.

[3] Michael Ortiz Hill, *Sacred Illness, Sacred Medicine* (Salt Lake City: Elik Press, 2005), 6–9.

[4] Michael Ortiz Hill and Deena Metzger, *Meeting Sacred Illness* (Salt Lake City: Elik Press, 2005), 7–8.

[5] Ibid., 26–27.

[6] Robert Bosnak, *A Little Course in Dreams* (Boston: Shambhala, 1998), 35.

The Imaginal Realm
of Dissociation

*The Archetypal Nature of Trauma
in Light of Quantum Physics*

JUDITH R. HARRIS

Many readers will surely recall the movie *Annie Hall* where the young boy Alvie is complaining of depression and is taken by his mother to a psychiatrist. After some prodding, the young boy finally tells the doctor what is wrong: "The universe is expanding," he says, "and if it is expanding, someday it will break apart and that will be the end of everything."

How can we understand this statement today in light of the new research on trauma and quantum physics from an archetypal perspective? Carl Gustav Jung and Wolfgang Pauli were pondering these questions fifty years ago, and yet in many ways the answers still remain a mystery.[1]

As we know, trauma is an experience of such overwhelming magnitude that the ego is in danger of being almost completely wiped out. Often the real danger lies in the fact that many severe traumas happen before the ego is fully formed—in other words, in the preverbal state when the human being is most fragile. Today, however, we have many advantages that Jung did not have, including brain-imaging techniques that are allowing us to actually see the physiological effects on the mind itself. Mind and body, or psyche and soma, are being brought together in an extraordinary way. We are dealing at a much more complex level than ever before in bringing together aspects of biology, neuroscience, physics, medicine, and symbolic language. In simpler language, we are bringing together the concrete physical world and the body with the metaphorical imagination and connecting them as the unified field of quantum physics that Pauli began to investigate so many years ago.

Coming back to our boy Alvie, how can we better understand his depression, or, as I prefer to call it, his *trauma* that was constellated by a realization that the universe is expanding? And indeed it is.

In the late 1920s, the American astronomer Edwin Hubble found scientific evidence that our nearby galaxies are actually receding away from us at zipping speeds, far beyond the human ability to comprehend. In fact, Hubble discovered something even more remarkable: He found that stars closer to us were moving away at a certain speed, but stars that were even more distant were moving away even faster, leading him to the startling conclusion that we are living in an expanding universe. This was a revolutionary discovery since previously it was thought that there were eight planets, that the earth circled around the sun, and that our solar system was at the center of the Milky Way. This new insight, however, quickly displaced us from the idea of living in the center of a static, stable, and secure universe and forced us to come to the startling realization that we are living in a dynamic, evolving world. We are reminded of the Buddhist who tells us that the only constant in life is change.

Staying with science for a moment, we also now know that throughout this expanding space swirling around at the time of creation, vast clouds of invisible nonatomic particles called dark matter collapsed under the force of their own gravity. These particles stuck together and formed what we call black holes. Contrary to what has previously been thought, black holes do not wipe out information that has been stored in matter; to our surprise, the information inside the black hole has not been lost at all! Instead we discover that it is actually stored holographically on the surface of the black hole itself. This statement becomes very important when we begin the difficult task of decoding traumatic memories that long ago were repressed somewhere in the vast unknown.

In addition to the realization that the universe we live in is expanding in runaway mode, we also face the prospect of becoming colder and darker as time progresses. If this were really to continue, it is possible that everything would freeze up, plunging us into the darkness of death. Is the annihilation that Alvie felt so threatening that he can no longer bear living out his life?

Traumatic experience almost always involves *dissociation*, the extent of which depends on the nature and the severity of the trauma. A standard medical dictionary defines dissociation as "an unconscious process by which a group of mental processes is separated from the rest of the thinking processes, resulting in an independent functioning of these processes and a loss of the usual relationships; for example, a separation of affect from cognition."[2] I would not hesitate to add here that dissociation is a violent act that comes as a consequence of severe psychological shock, which very often seriously impairs integrative functions. Trauma ruptures the personality into what Jung called autonomous splinter psyches,[3] which become split off as a result of these overwhelming traumatic experiences. Trauma shatters innocence for, as one author describes it, "when innocence has been deprived of its entitlement, it becomes a diabolical spirit."[4]

Dissociation is an explosion that is forced tyrannically upon us against our conscious will. It causes a shattering of the whole, sending the fragmented pieces out away from the center. We must never forget, however, that dissociation can often allow for a sense of safety in the individual concerned. Without it, a complete shattering of the psyche could occur. As with all entities in the archetypal world, dissociation has two sides: first, the horrific and unthinkable; and second, the element of protection it provides against the possibility of the psyche's breaking apart into individual components, leaving the individual in a severe state of fragmentation. Some of the associated symptoms of dissociation include a feeling of leaving one's body and a sense of detachment, moments of losing track or blanking out, finding oneself acting on automatic pilot without conscious awareness of one's actions, feelings of floating or levitation, and loss of bodily sensations or, in some cases, numbing of pain altogether. These are just a few consequences of this shattering of the vessel, as I call it—in other words, the breaking apart of the vessel as container. Or, metaphorically speaking, the paradisiacal situation has been overthrown. But to what avail?

It is imperative that the healing of trauma be taken to the depths of archetypal experience in order to repair the symbolic capacity that is so often damaged in these patients. Is it possible to find a solution for Alvie so that all or some of his anxiety can be alleviated?

Here we ask what may seem an obvious question: Is there a difference between what happens in the outer world around us as opposed to what we experience in the inner world? In other words, is there a difference between what we experience imaginatively and what appears to us in concrete form? These are absolutely imperative questions since not only is our conference entitled *Imagination and Medicine* but without imagination, where would we be? Would we not be trapped in a world of causality, nothing buts, and superficialities? Albert Einstein once remarked, "Imagination is more important than knowledge."[5]

Long before Einstein the medieval alchemists were aware that they were working with the imagination as they projected their unconscious onto matter. In fact, the alchemists were not only relating to the unconscious, they were relating directly to the substance they were hoping to transform, solely through the power of the imagination. More than any other power, imagination is what distinguishes the human psyche; it is human existence itself. In his volume *Psychology and Alchemy*,[6] therefore, Jung says that the imagination is a concentrated extract of the life force, meaning, of course, both in the psychic and physical senses. Imagination, we learn, is the faculty that frees us from static images and transforms them.

With our previous conception of trauma, we must find a new attitude that will, above all, incorporate the healing factor inherent at the archetypal core. After all, the archetype, as Jung discovered, is the deposit of all human experience right back to its remotest beginnings. As the archetype is our store of energy and, therefore, indestructible, one feels reinforced, strengthened. Archetypes cannot be changed, but, as Jung tells us, they can be refined and developed according to the present culture and history of the moment. They are eternal, they live in our unconscious, and it is our task, therefore, to make the unconscious conscious; in other words, to use the archetypal healing factor in the service of allowing energy to change thoughts and images and experience healing at this profound, meaningful level.

Is it possible to once again look at the image of our boy Alvie and to feel his distress upon coming to the realization that the world is indeed expanding and that one day it may very well no longer be in existence? What has thus far been safe and secure for him, or at least to some degree, is evidently no longer so, and it is as if the certainties of his world are slipping away. Leaving paradise is never an easy task, but it is a sacrifice that must be undertaken if we are not to remain in an infantile state in which neither relationship nor creativity is possible. We can revel in the natural unconsciousness that paradise offers us—and perhaps we think of life in this way before a devastating trauma comes upon us. Unfortunately, however, the majority of the very serious traumas we encounter are those that happen long before the fullness of time, so to speak—long before the ego forms or far too often long before the ego has even a chance to form into a nascent being. We are speaking here of preverbal trauma, and I believe that research in healing these extremely difficult and all-too-common cases is just beginning. In Jungian terms we must say, therefore, that somehow and in some way this horrific event comes to us for some reason, some inexplicable reason that we cannot yet understand from the ego point of view. Destiny must somehow be reckoned with. In many instances it seems so unfair, so devastating, yet the only meaningful way to comprehend it is to see it as an impetus towards healing, as Jung called it—a *gradient*, or movement, toward wholeness.

Our boy Alvie is caught in the archetypal agony of being in exile, not only from his own personal circumstances but from the world around him as well. He is petrified of annihilation and of the threatened dissolution of his so-called coherent self, as Kohut calls it.[7] His center has, for some unknown reason, been shaken. We are left only to conjecture what the explanation could possibly be, but in the film we are given the impression that the answer is not so simple but rather a complex conglomeration of factors, not precluding primal attachment pathologies. The Jungian analyst Donald Kalsched explains that to experience such anxiety actually threatens the total extinction of the human personality and consequently the destruction of the human spirit.[8]

Over and over again we see in various myths from around the world that the creative process begins with the breaking apart of opposites. Creation can only take place in the space formed by their separation. Chaos must separate out into thousands of pieces, so to speak, in order for consciousness to be born. When the earth and the heavens were separated from each other in the first chapter of Genesis, for example, light and darkness became differentiated from one another. We live in that space between, the space that quantum physics tells us is teeming with possibilities. In Kabbalistic myth it is said that God had to contract himself, an act of self-retraction, in order to make space for creation, for the human realm.[9] The urge to create is what brought the life force into being.

In Genesis 1:1 it is said that "darkness covered the face of the waters." Later in the Old Testament, in the book of Isaiah, it is said, "I form the light, and create darkness; I make peace, and create evil; I am the Lord, that doeth all these things."[10] With the creation of life, initiated by the withdrawal of divine energy—in other words, through the sacrifice of the divine in favour of the human world—evil enters, as the one-sidedness of divine luminosity gives way to the world of reality. In Kabbalistic thought, this newly-created space can generate worlds, worlds brought about by exile from the original unity. Mistakenly we can find ourselves in an empty concrete world, devoid of hope or faith.

Or we can recall the line by Wallace Stevens: "And not to have is the beginning of desire."[11]

Is not the exile from original unity our archetypal journey that cannot be escaped? Is it not true that all being has been in exile since the very beginning of creation? Exile, by its very nature, erodes the sense of self and the connections between self and world. After all, the first most important phase in the life of Abraham begins when he is told by God, "Go forth from your native land, from your birthplace, and from your father's house to the land that I will show you."[12] We are reminded here that wandering in exile has an archetypal, divine purpose and that is to gather up the sparks that have been scattered throughout the cosmos. This inner fragmentation that so petrifies Alvie in the film mirrors his view of the world, which he sees as a multitude of separate objects and events. The belief that all these separate parts really do exist and live in isolation has served to alienate us from ourselves, from our fellow human beings, and from the world.

I will take us further by boldly suggesting that trauma is an archetypal happening that shatters the original unity and sends sparks—in other words, dissociated fragments from the existing whole—out into the universe, often so far away that the contents feel almost irretrievable. I further propose that the origin of the universe we are living in began with such a cataclysmic explosion, referred to as the Big Bang, which sent the stars and galaxies hurtling outward into space. Scientists are even suggesting that this action of creating the universe is happening every split second as we speak, that it was not a one-time occurrence but rather a constant repetition of cosmology. It is speculated that there actually was a collection of dots that appeared shortly after the Big Bang and that these dots represent fluctuations or irregularities from the original, primal state. These tiny fluctuations are like seeds that have since grown and expanded enormously as the universe itself exploded outward. Today, these tiny seeds have blossomed into the galactic clusters that we see lighting up the heavens. In this scenario, which quantum scientists have named the inflationary theory, in the first trillionth of a trillionth of a second a mysterious antigravity force caused the universe to expand actually much faster than the speed of light.

We can think of the antigravity force as that force that pulls us out of reality and away from the ground when we dissociate, and which takes us out of our bodies and may even put us into a trance-like state in order to take us away from the pain of an overwhelming, traumatic event. Incidentally, we are not violating Einstein's theory that says that nothing can travel faster than the speed of light since it is empty space in this case that is expanding. Within a fraction of a second, in the inflationary theory of the cosmos, the universe expanded by an unimaginable factor of 10^{50}. It has even been suggested that universes may be continually giving birth to new universes. If this is true, we are living in a sea of multiverses, or many universes. Is this cosmological theory able to help us in our treatment of trauma?

Let us come back for a moment to the spaces or gaps between the dissociated fragments in the traumatic experience. How can we begin to understand them in the new paradigm of the twenty-first century? One man in my analytic practice described the gap as a place of intolerable anxiety when he is forced to spend a night away from his wife. Another analysand described this gap as a place where she "dumped all the trash of life," a place where she has found it easy to live only half a life. Yet another woman told me recently that there is always a gap between herself and her husband, that something is missing, that there seems to be no real connection at the soul level. Another woman, severely traumatized from repeated early sexual assault, told me not long ago that she always lives in the gap, that real life has not yet touched her. This particular woman says that in this gap her trauma lives, taking her in and out of memories and keeping her out of her body and out of the real world around her. Where are we actually when we are in the gap?

More than fifty years ago, Carl Gustav Jung was attempting to bring the mind and body together in a meaningful way. What is often forgotten, however, is that what Jung was actually most interested

in was the space that serves as the connector between these two seemingly opposing worlds. Jung described this very carefully in a paper
entitled "On the Nature of the Psyche":

> Since psyche and matter are contained in one and the same
> world, and moreover are in continuous contact with one an-
> other and ultimately rest on irrepresentable factors, it is not only
> possible but fairly probable, even, that psyche and matter are
> two different aspects of one and the same thing. The
> synchronicity phenomena point, it seems to me, in this direc-
> tion, for they show that the nonpsychic can behave like the
> psychic, and vice versa, without there being any causal connec-
> tion between them. Our present knowledge does not allow us
> to do much more than compare the relation of the psychic to
> the material world with two cones, whose apices, meeting in a
> point without extension—a real zero-point—touch and don't
> touch.[13]

This is the place in-between, of the gap, so to speak, the place we
often refer to as the subtle body, the intermediate place between spirit
and body and between the heavenly and earthly realms. It is here that
body and spirit are united as one and have a mutual influence on each
other. It is a crossing-over between the divine and human worlds, the place
where image and symbol serve as connectors between the two realms. It
is here that neuroscience seems to have an ability to take us further.

Coming back to the zero-point that Jung writes about in this
passage, we must seriously ask ourselves what this could really mean.
It seems to have been left in a very mysterious way since Jung, as he
admits himself, could not take this image any further, due simply to
the lack of scientific knowledge at that time. Remember, we are speaking about more than fifty years ago. Today we have the ability to begin a new journey because quantum science has discovered the zero-
point field.

What could this zero-point field consist of that Jung was investigating all these years ago? Quantum physicists have discovered an
ocean of microscopic vibrations that exist in the space between things.
They have realized that the very underpinning of our universe is in
fact a heaving sea of energy. These scientists began to speculate that if
this indeed is true, then everything is connected to everything else,
like some mysterious invisible web. In fact, modern science has now
demonstrated that there is no such thing as pure nothingness, that a

vacuum is full of zero-point energy. This field is termed to be zero because fluctuations within this field are still detectable at temperatures of absolute zero, which is the lowest possible energy state, wherein all matter has supposedly been removed and nothing is left that can make motion possible. Zero-point energy is the energy present in this emptiest of space at the lowest possible point of energy. Furthermore, the physicists also tell us that it is not possible to bring anything completely to rest, that there will in fact always be a minuscule amount of movement present at any time. These gaps, which we experience in the dissociated traumatic experience, are pregnant, therefore, with thoughts, emotions, bodily sensations, and so on. Our challenge is to connect *into* the field, allowing the healing factor to be constellated in this vast sea of huge dynamic energy. Scientific evidence for Jung's premise of the subtle body is coming to the fore.

It appears that the zero-point field allows these subatomic molecules to communicate with each other in vast ways. We now have evidence that these fragmentations of thought and emotion are always connected one way or another, *no matter what*. In addition, at some level the imprint of our ancestral, biological, and cognitive memories lies in this ocean of space along with all our possibilities for the future, and it connects the future with the past and with the present, bringing the timeless, spaceless archetypal world into reality within and without.

Psychologists have been describing this potential space for a long time, in particular the British psychoanalyst D.W. Winnicott, who called it the intermediate area where we *experience* and a place where inner and outer reality meet *in relationship*. In Winnicott's terms, it also encompasses the paradox of standing alone yet being in the presence of someone else. Is this not the profound mystical state many of us have been searching for? Winnicott speaks of this place of union in which everything can happen as a place where the arts, religion, all imaginative living, and in fact all creativity belongs. In the beginning, as with all creation, there is the original unity of mother and baby where at first there is (or ideally so) virtually no separation between mother and child, and this develops through various phases into two separate, yet interrelated beings. Trust becomes an absolute prerequisite for the enjoyment of what Winnicott so aptly called relaxation, the place where surrender takes the place of rigidity and a compulsion to control, pathologies too often seen in our world today.

To repeat, these spaces that are created and involuntarily fly out at incomprehensible speeds to unknown far-flung places in that moment in which trauma occurs, and tragically often reoccurs, often become the places that are teeming with creative possibilities.

A woman came to see me some years ago with a severe repeated history of trauma since her early life. What was unusual about this woman, however, was her uncanny ability to work with her own material and to stand back, almost objectively, from it. Her capacity to go in and out of the traumas, so to speak, not always at will but often with barely any prompting, gives us a wealth of material from which to draw. In addition, she was an artist, which gave her from an early age an immense connection to the archetypal world. I will call her Susan.

Susan had thus far managed her life quite well. When she was a young girl at school her teachers often complained that she would daydream far too much and later when she came into analysis, she had an awareness that her life was only half lived, threatened with dissolution at any time. An unexpected turn in her life threw her into what she called heaving traumas, in which her body literally went into convulsions as she was thrown in and out of unbearable psychic states. Having lived in an unsatisfactory marriage for many years, Susan began an extramarital affair that she described as the biggest life-changing event that had ever happened to her. It felt to her as if the man, himself also married, was the catalyst who was meant to change her entire life. Unexpectedly, however, from what seemed like one day to the next, this man began to pull away and soon admitted a sudden change of mind—that in reality he was not going to leave his own marriage and go away with her. In fact, he even began to act coldly to her at times, which sent Susan into periods of uncontrollable crying that often went on for days. The devastation was far too much to bear, and she began having such overwhelming symptoms that work became difficult and almost impossible. At this point she came into analysis with me.

Early on in our work together, Susan wrote in her journal: "anxiety of falling, falling must come from infancy." Somehow she already knew the truth. Her mother became ill with cancer when she was very young, and after a period of many years of bedridden illness, she finally died when Susan was nine years old. This man became to her the mother she never had, and his withholding of the nurturing she had initially experienced at the start of their relationship constellated all her early traumas, concerning which space does not permit me to go into here.

In her relationship with this man, Susan was flung, almost violently, between the opposites, floundering in deep, early trauma. Fortunately, I was able to rely on the work pioneered by Marion Woodman, bringing the psyche-body connection that Jung wrote about so many years ago to fruition.[14]

Coming back once again to Jung's zero-point, the points between that "touch and don't touch," the place connecting the opposites of psyche and body—spirit and matter, psyche and soma, or instinct and archetype, as they may also be called—we come across something quite extraordinary: Neuroscience has actually begun to see this zero-point field, the void, often called the vacuum, as the place we have previously spoken of where nothingness transforms into everything and as the science of love, the place of possibilities, of connection in relationship. Could bodywork, or, I should rather say, conscious bodywork, literally transform the early imprints deep in the cells of our bodies, touching the subtle body at the archetypal level?

Turning once again to neuroscience, we may indeed find some clues to questions that have been asked for decades. Recent developments begin to provide us with an empirical understanding of how to work with patients like Susan and of how to further the work of Carl Jung and Wolfgang Pauli in their investigations into the workings of the unconscious from a scientific point of view. It is becoming increasingly clear that the development of consciousness is essentially a relational process. Jung wrote in his *Psychology of the Transference* that the bond between doctor and patient is of mutual benefit. In other words, as he said, "when two chemical substances combine, both are altered." Every advance in treatment, from the perspective of neuroscience, involves both participants in an essential way.

We recall that Susan came into analysis because of a desperate feeling of falling, an experience which she knew somehow must come from infancy. Winnicott describes this feeling as "unthinkable anxiety" and lack of relationship to the body.[15] In 1962, he wrote that all babies are actually on the brink of unthinkable anxiety and that the only way to stave off this unbearable psychic state is for the mother to be "good enough" and to be able to meet the needs of her infant in what we might call a reasonably adequate way. Winnicott says further that the only way for a mother to show love at this crucial early stage is through the care of her little one's body.[16]

In the BodySoul workshops originally developed by Marion Woodman, Mary Hamilton, and Ann Skinner,[17] we try to recreate through various exercises the original condition of the ideal state between mother and child. We return once again to alchemical symbolism in which the goal of the process is to return the body to its original state, to the form at the beginning of the *opus*, at the time of creation. It is very likely that the dissociative response to trauma is expressed as it was first experienced in the spectrum of the psyche-soma relationship. Conflicts that are not able to withstand the pain of consciousness are liable to be stored in body memory. The more experience we have with histories of trauma, the more we learn that we must take the body into full account.

From neuroscience we have learned that imagination, thought, memory, and feeling all take place in the spaces between our nerve cells in synaptic transmission. Synapses are the tiny gaps between neurons that, in communicating various messages throughout the brain, actually close the gap, helping us to function as integrated individuals. Dissociation can serve to break these vital links, thereby fragmenting and alienating us from society and from ourselves. It has been found that it is possible for adults to increase their neural connections by learning new ways of being in the world and in relation to others. Through the embodiment of repeated positive experiences, for example, it may very well be possible not only to strengthen existing neural connections but also to grow entirely new synapses, thereby increasing the integrative capacity of brain and emotional functioning.

It is clear that trauma needs to be undone in both the mind and the body. We come back once again to the gap, to the space which lies between dissociated fragments in a traumatic experience, to the space between the psychic and instinctual realms, to the synapse, the space which transmits the chemical messengers to various sites throughout the body, and, last, to the limbic system, that part of our brain in which raw emotion is generated and alarm bells are switched on in traumatic states. In each of these cases, the space between signifies a connector between opposite modes of experience. Jung referred to this place of connection as a symbol, as a metaphor which brings a healing factor into reality. In fact, neuroscience has been looking at the role of metaphor in facilitating memory recall in traumatic dissociation because of metaphor's ability to reestablish the collaboration of both the right and left hemispheres in the aftermath of trauma.

My patient, Susan, is in the process of deep healing of her early traumas. Our relationship has been a key factor in the transformation, allowing both bodywork and dream work to touch at the deep cellular level. Gradually memories have been surfacing, and somehow during this journey it has become clear that when we reach into one traumatic memory, it is as if all traumatic memories begin to collide with one another in what we might call a chaotic mess. Space limitations do not permit me to go further into chaos theory here, but we may remember Nietzsche saying: "One must still have chaos in one, to give birth to a dancing star."[18]

Once again, quantum theory helps us in the treatment of these acute and unthinkable psychic states. According to quantum theorists, the most bizarre aspect of the quantum world is the phenomenon we call entanglement. Entangled entities, or, fragments of thought, body memories, or flashbacks are linked together in the unconscious because they are produced in some similar way to each other. These pieces apparently fly off in all directions, as Alvie experienced in his perception of the expanding universe, yet quantum theory tells us that while two particles, most often opposing tendencies such as hot and cold, can seem very far apart, even millions of miles away from each other, they are actually linked together in some mysterious and uncanny way. And, furthermore, what happens to one of these fragments *simultaneously* causes a change in the other. The fact that this change is instantaneous accounts for synchronistic quantum leaps that are paramount in the spontaneous healings described in the literature. It seems that these fragmented pieces are not lost at all, that in fact they search for union with each other in an almost mystical re-union.

In conclusion, it is clear, therefore, that dissociation impairs the unified sense of self that we all yearn for. Jung makes this abundantly clear when he writes:

> A dissociation is not healed by being split off, but by more complete disintegration. All the powers that strive for unity, all healthy desire for selfhood, will resist the disintegration, and in this way [the analysand] will become conscious of the possibility of an inner integration, which before he had always sought

outside himself. He will then find his reward in an undivided self.[19]

Bringing together trauma theory and quantum mechanics in the space between the opposites reminds me of what Rainer Maria Rilke said when he came upon Brancusi's sculpture, *Bird in Space:* "After this, we will all have to live a little differently."[20]

NOTES

[1] For more information, see David Lindorff, *Pauli and Jung* (Wheaton, IL: Quest Books, 2004) and J. Gary Sparks, *At The Heart of Matter* (Toronto: Inner City Books, 2007).

[2] *Stedman's Medical Dictionary: Twenty-fourth Edition* (Baltimore: Williams & Wilkins, 1982), 416, quoted in Robert C. Scaer, *The Body Bears The Burden: Trauma, Dissociation, and Disease* (Binghamton, NY: The Haworth Medical Press, 2001), 19.

[3] See C. G. Jung, "A Review of the Complex Theory," *The Structure and Dynamics of the Psyche,* trans. R. F. C. Hull, vol. 8 of *The Collected Works of C. G. Jung* (Princeton, NJ: Princeton Univ. Press, 1960), § 204; hereafter abbreviated as *CW* followed by volume number and paragraph (§) number.

[4] Grotstein, J., "Forgery of the Soul," in C. Nelson and M. Eigen (eds.), *Evil, Self and Culture* (New York: Human Sciences Press, 1984), 203–26, quoted in Donald Kalsched, *The Inner World of Trauma* (New York: Routledge, 1996), 11.

[5] Walter Isaacson, *Einstein: His Life and Universe* (New York: Simon & Schuster, 2007), 7.

[6] C. G. Jung, *Psychology and Alchemy, CW* 12.

[7] Heinz Kohut, *The Analysis of the Self* (New York: International Universities Press, 1971).

[8] Donald Kalsched, *The Inner World of Trauma*, 1.

[9] See Judith Harris, *Jung and Yoga: The Psyche-Body Connection* (Toronto: Inner City Books, 2001), 111.

[10] Isaiah 45:7.

[11] Wallace Stevens, "Notes Toward a Supreme Fiction," *Collected Poetry and Prose* (New York: The Library of America, 1972), 330.

[12] Genesis 12:1.

[13] C. G. Jung, "On the Nature of the Psyche," *CW 8* § 418.

¹⁴ See, for example, Marion Woodman, *The Pregnant Virgin* (Toronto: Inner City Books, 1985), 62f.

¹⁵D. W. Winnicott, *Playing and Reality* (New York and London: Routledge, 1991), 97.

¹⁶D. W. Winnicott, *Ego Integration in Child Development* (London: Tavistock Publications, 1962).

¹⁷ See *Spring 72, Body and Soul: Honoring Marion Woodman* (New Orleans, LA: Spring Journal, 2005).

¹⁸ C. G. Jung, *Seminar on Nietzsche's Zarathustra* (Princeton: Princeton University Press, 1988), 105.

¹⁹ C. G. Jung, "Marriage as a Psychological Relationship," *CW 17* § 334.

²⁰ Leonard Shlain, *Art & Physics* (New York: HarperCollins, 1991), 363.

Science

5

Can Believing Make You Well? A Decade Later

ESTHER M. STERNBERG, M.D.

As I sit by my friend's bedside in the fading afternoon light of a cloudy day, I hear the steady click of the intravenous pump, alternating with the ticking of the large clock on the wall across her bed. Below the clock is a daily calendar showing the day and date and year—the kind that you can rip off page-by-page, day-by-day, like in the old Hollywood movies that show time flying by. In big silver letters it announces: "*Today is*" and under that is a huge shadowed *27*; below that: *Wednesday, August 2008*. The nurses' voices are muffled on the other side of the thick wooden door. The stillness is occasionally interrupted by a loud intercom's *brreep* followed by a human voice calling out a name and number or instruction. My friend's breathing is calm—barely discernable by the gentle rise and fall of her chest. She seems so peaceful there asleep.

I think back to a similar hospital room, over a decade ago, where my mother lay, where I sat typing on another laptop—one much clunkier and bigger then than the light, file-folder thin one that now sits balanced on my thigh. The armchair then was in the same spot in the room relative to the bed as the one on which I now sit, off to her left and up against the window. My mother had the same illness as my friend has now. She had had surgery to remove a mass on the same side—the left, in the same breast, and lymph nodes under the same arm. But it was not August 27, 2008. Had a wall calendar announced the date, it would have read *January 1997*.

In that decade so much has changed. My mother's cancer was not caught early, as my friend's has been. By the time the surgeon's knife had cut into my mother's breast, the tumor had already spread. There were two large masses, and the lymph nodes had already sucked up their share of tumor cells. It was six years from the time of diagnosis in 1991 before my mother finally succumbed, with many hospital visits in between. It was in those final days when I sat beside her bed and wrote the *Scientific American* article that later became the book from which the following chapter is reprinted.

The sensitive MRI imaging technique that detected my friend's cancer was just being perfected back then: the kind that relies on magnetic fields to paint a sharp and detailed image of the breast, normal tissue and diseased, so that cancer cells can be detected before they spread. Back then, the images were still fuzzy, out of focus compared to what we can see now. The treatments too are so much better now. The cuts from the surgeon's knife are much smaller; the radiation more focused; the chemotherapy more powerful and specific and with less nausea and vomiting. All this has resulted in much longer remission times and even cures. The attitudes and rules of the hospital have changed too—the staff understands the importance of family and friends in the healing process. The first thing the nurse said to me as she ushered me into my friend's hospital room was "There are no visiting hours here—you can come and go anytime you like." The chair in which I sat pulled out into a sofa bed, so I could stay all night.

But one thing has not changed at all: the patient's faith and hope in healing. My friend's deep and abiding faith has seen her this far in the process and will continue to guide her as she moves forward, through the immediate post-op pain, through dealing with the draining pump, through the reconstruction, through physiotherapy, all the way to the other side. The night before the surgery, a friend sent her two quotes from the Scriptures, which she downloaded, printed out, and carried with her, tightly clutched, into the operating room. One was from Jeremiah, the other from Isaiah:

> Jer 17:14 Heal me, O LORD, and I shall be healed; save me,
> and I shall be saved: for thou [art] my praise.

> Isa 53:5 But he [was] wounded for our transgressions, [he was]
> bruised for our iniquities: the chastisement of our peace [was]
> upon him; and with his stripes we are healed.

No matter how far back we reach into human history and experience, faith and prayer have been tightly linked to healing.

The last time I sat like this, beside my mother's bed in the quiet
of a fading afternoon, I did not believe that believing could make you
well. I myself had not yet experienced my own set of illnesses. In that
cocky, self-assured way that academic physicians learn, I sneered then
at that notion, even though I had studied the science of the mind-
body connection. I was skeptical, even though in my work in the lab
I had literally touched the very part of the brain that controls the stress
response: the hypothalamus. I criticized the idea that belief could heal,
even though I had measured the brain's stress hormones in patients
and could see their effects on the immune system in real time.

What I sat writing on those afternoons beside my mother's bed
in 1997 was an article for the *Scientific American* on the science of the
mind-body connection. It mainly focused on the brain's stress response
and how stress could make you sick. In the paper, I carefully avoided
the topic of belief and the possible effect of salubrious activities, like
prayer and meditation, on healing. But my mother disagreed. She
mostly dozed, but when she intermittently awoke, she quizzed me
on what I was writing.

I described to her how during chronic stress, the brain's stress
center, the hypothalamus, pumps out its hormones, which in turn
cause the adrenal glands to pump out cortisol—a hormone necessary
for life, for energy to fight or flee from danger. I told her how stress
can also suppress the immune system, making one prone to infections,
slowing wound healing and lowering take-rate to vaccines. My mother
argued that this was all well and good, but what about belief? What
about the benefits of quiet, peaceful times, like when she worked in
her garden? What about prayer? I countered that there was no solid
scientific evidence for any of that, and so I had no plans to include
those concepts in the article. And so I did not. The article focused on
stress and illness, not on belief and healing. After my mother died,
when I wrote the proposal for the book that became *The Balance Within*,
I planned to debunk the notion that believing could make you well.
But that was then and this is now.

As I wrote the chapter that is excerpted here, I found that even at the end of the 1990s there was accumulating evidence to show not only that believing could make you well but also how it could do so. The scientific term for this phenomenon is called the "placebo effect." It is an unfortunate term because it carries with it negative associations that have grown out of decades of lack of understanding of the power and nature of this effect. The phrase is often preceded by the word "just," as in: "just the placebo effect"—implying that this is a biologically meaningless effect, something to be subtracted out from the biological effect of a "real" cure. But placebo and the brain's placebo mechanisms are very real. They are in fact the brain and body's own self-healing mechanisms.

A decade ago there were already pharmacological data showing that the brain's endogenous opiate pathways—those nerves that pump out pain-numbing chemicals, the endorphins—are activated during the placebo effect. Release of such chemicals during pain can truly help to numb pain. The trick is to find the ways to trigger that release when it is needed. There was also evidence to show that a kind of learning called conditioning might come into play during the placebo effect. But that was about as far as it went. It was these aspects of placebo, its historical roots and the scientists and their scientific discoveries that I describe in the chapter that follows.

In the decade since I wrote that chapter, enormous strides have been made in understanding the placebo effect and the brain mechanisms that are activated during the state we call belief. Many of these, made by researchers at the forefront of the field, are described in other chapters in this volume. These include activation of not only the endogenous opiate pathways but also of the brain's dopamine reward pathways. During states of belief, whether through prayer or meditation or simply believing that a saltwater solution is an active drug, the brain releases chemicals that numb pain and other chemicals that trigger desire and satisfaction. We know this because brain-imaging studies using radioactive-labeled opiate or dopamine-like chemicals have shown activation of receptors for these nerve chemicals during placebo conditions. Some researchers have even measured the electrical activity of single nerve cells in the reward regions of the brain in patients undergoing brain surgery. These studies show that nerve cells' electrical activity changes in patients whose symptoms improve when treated with a placebo but does not change in patients in whom there is no improvement. Other researchers have shown that many of these same brain regions are also activated during states of meditation and prayer.

We now have a much better understanding of how activation of such brain systems can influence the immune system through the brain's outflow pathways, which are also shifted during such states. Researchers have shown that the adrenalin stress response, which kicks the heart and blood pressure into high gear, downshifts into a relaxation pattern—one governed by the nerve chemical acetylcholine, released by the vagus nerve during such states. Practices like yoga, Tai Chi, or even moderate exercise make the variability of the heart's rhythms increase, telling us that the stress response has shifted towards the relaxation response. Much of this is triggered by breathing—the slow and rhythmic breathing that practitioners of yoga are trained to do. But other repetitive patterns can also help us achieve such states: repeated words of prayer or mantras, like rosary prayer or Buddhist chants; visualizing images; or thinking about compassion. Regular moderate exercise also enhances positive brain pathways, including dopamine reward and serotonin systems. Finally, research is accumulating that shows that enhancement of these brain regions and pathways also strengthens the immune system and helps protect against those negative effects of chronic stress on illness.

Much work remains to be done, but the path is clear. There is now no question that the answer to the question I posed a decade ago in the chapter that follows—"Can Believing Make You Well?"—is a resounding yes. We are learning more each day about how this works. In so doing we can all feel confident that by incorporating these techniques and approaches into our daily lives, we will not only reduce the negative effects of stress but also enhance the positive, and ultimately help maintain wellness.

ADDITIONAL READING

Neurobiology of Placebo

de la Fuente-Fernandez, R., M. Schulzer et al. "Placebo Mechanisms and Reward Circuitry: Clues From Parkinson's Disease." *Biol Psychiatry* 56(2) (2004): 67–71.

de la Fuente-Fernandez, R., and A. J. Stoessl. "The Biochemical Bases of the Placebo Effect." *Sci Eng Ethics* 10(1) (2004): 143–50.

Finniss, D. G., and F. Benedetti. "Mechanisms of the Placebo Response and Their Impact on Clinical Trials and Clinical Practice." *Pain* 114(1–2) (2005): 3–6.

Lanotte, M., L. Lopiano et al. "Expectation Enhances Autonomic Responses to Stimulation of the Human Subthalamic Limbic Region." *Brain Behav Immun* 19(6) (2005): 500–9.

Levine, J. D., N. C. Gordon et al. "The Mechanism of Placebo Analgesia." *Lancet* 2(8091) (1978): 654–7.

Levine, J. D., N. C. Gordon et al. "Naloxone Dose Dependently Produces Analgesia and Hyperalgesia in Postoperative Pain." *Nature* 278(5706) (1979): 740–1.

Stewart-Williams, S., and J. Podd. "The Placebo Effect: Dissolving the Expectancy Versus Conditioning Debate." *Psychol Bull* 130(2) (2004): 324–40.

Wager, T. D., J. K. Rilling et al. "Placebo-induced Changes in FMRI in the Anticipation and Experience of Pain." *Science* 303(5661) (2004): 1162–7.

Zubieta, J. K., Y. R. Smith et al. "Regional Mu Opioid Receptor Regulation of Sensory and Affective Dimensions of Pain." *Science* 293(5528) (2001): 311–5.

Neurobiology of Meditation

Barinaga, M. . "Buddhism and Neuroscience. Studying the Well-trained Mind." *Science* 302(5642) (2003): 44–6.

Brefczynski-Lewis, J. A., A. Lutz et al. . "Neural Correlates of Attentional Expertise in Long-term Meditation Practitioners." *Proc Natl Acad Sci U S A* 104(27) (2007): 11483–8.

Lutz, A., L. L. Greischar et al. "Long-term Meditators Self-induce High-amplitude Gamma Synchrony During Mental Practice." *Proc Natl Acad Sci U S A* 101(46) (2004): 16369–73.

Melloni, L., C. Molina et al. "Synchronization of Neural Activity Across Cortical Areas Correlates with Conscious Perception." *J Neurosci* 27(11) (2007): 2858–65.

Davidson, R. J., J. Kabat-Zinn et al. "Alterations in Brain and Immune Function Produced by Mindfulness Meditation." *Psychosom Med* 65(4) (2003): 564–70.

Lutz, A., J. Brefczynski-Lewis et al. "Regulation of the Neural Circuitry of Emotion by Compassion Meditation: Effects of Meditative Expertise." *PLoS ONE* 3(3) (2008): e1897.

Lutz, A., H. A. Slagter et al. "Attention Regulation and Monitoring in Meditation." *Trends Cogn Sci* 12(4) (2008): 163–9.

Peng, C. K., I. C. Henry et al. "Heart Rate Dynamics During Three Forms of Meditation." *Int J Cardiol.* 95(1) (2004): 19–27.

Neurobiology of Prayer

Beauregard, M., and V. Paquette. "Neural Correlates of a Mystical Experience in Carmelite Nuns." *Neurosci Lett* 405(3) (2006): 186–90.

Newberg, A., M. Pourdehnad et al. "Cerebral Blood Flow During Meditative Prayer: Preliminary Findings and Methodological Issues." *Percept Mot Skills* 97(2) (2003): 625–30.

Exercise: Effects on Neuroplasticity, Mood, Immune System and Health

Brown, J. D., and J. M. Siegel . "Exercise as a Buffer of Life Stress: A Prospective Study of Adolescent Health." *Health Psychol* 7(4) (1988): 341–53.

Dishman, R. K., H. R. Berthoud et al. "Neurobiology of Exercise." *Obesity* (Silver Spring) 14(3) (2006): 345–56.

Duman, R. S.. "Neurotrophic Factors and Regulation of Mood: Role of Exercise, Diet and Metabolism." *Neurobiol Aging* 26 Suppl 1 (2005): 88–93.

Foley, T. E., and M. Fleshner. "Neuroplasticity of Dopamine Circuits After Exercise: Implications for Central Fatigue." *Neuromolecular Med.* (2008).

Greenwood, B. N., T. E. Foley et al. "The Consequences of Uncontrollable Stress are Sensitive to Duration of Prior Wheel Running." *Brain Res* 1033(2) (2005): 164–78.

Yeung, R. R. "The Acute Effects of Exercise on Mood State." *J Psychosom Res* 40(2) (1996): 123–41.

Physiology of Tai Chi and Yoga

West, J., C. Otte et al. "Effects of Hatha Yoga and African Dance on Perceived Stress, Affect, and Salivary Cortisol." *Ann Behav Med* 28(2) (2004): 114–8.

Yeh, G. Y., J. E. Mietus et al. "Enhancement of Sleep Stability with Tai Chi Exercise in Chronic Heart Failure: Preliminary Findings Using an ECG-based Spectrogram Method." *Sleep Med.* (2007).

Yeh, G. Y., M. J. Wood et al. "Effects of Tai Chi Mind-Body Movement Therapy on Functional Status and Exercise Capacity in Patients with Chronic Heart Failure: A Randomized Controlled Trial." *Am J Med* 117(8) (2004): 541–8.

Brain-Immune Connection

Heijnen, C. J. "Who Believes in 'Communication'"? The Norman Cousins Lecture, 1999." *Brain Behav Immun* 14(1) (2000): 2–9.

Kuis, W., C. de Jong-de Vos van Steenwijk et al. "The Autonomic Nervous System and the Immune System in Juvenile Rheumatoid Arthritis." *Brain Behav Immun* 10(4) (1996): 387–98.

Marques-Deak, A., G. Cizza, and E. M. Sternberg. "Brain-immune Interactions and Disease Susceptibility." *Mol Psychiatry* 10 (3) (2005): 239–250.

Sanders, V. M. "Interdisciplinary Research: Noradrenergic Regulation of Adaptive Immunity." *Brain Behav Immun* 20(1) (2006): 1–8.

Sternberg, E. M. *The Balance Within: The Science Connecting Health and Emotions.* New York: W. H. Freeman, 2000 (hard cover); New York: Holt, Times Imprint, 2001 (paperback).

Sternberg, E. M., and P. W. Gold. "The Mind-Body Interaction in Disease." *Scientific American Special Edition: The Hidden Mind.* 12 (1) (2002): 82–89.

Sternberg, E. M.. "Neural Regulation of Innate Immunity: A Coordinated Nonspecific Host Response to Pathogens." *Nature Rev. Immunol.* 6(4) (2006): 318–28.

Webster, J. I., L. Tonelli, and E. M. Sternberg. "Neuroendocrine Regulation of Immunity." *Annual Rev Immunol* 20 (2002): 125–163.

Stress and Illness

Cohen, S., D. Janicki-Deverts et al. "Psychological Stress and Disease." *JAMA* 298(14) (2007): 1685–7.

Cohen, S., D. A. Tyrrell et al. "Psychological Stress and Susceptibility to the Common Cold." *New England Journal of Medicine* 325(9) (1991): 606–12.

Esterling, B. A., J. K. Kiecolt-Glaser et al. "Chronic Stress, Social Support, and Persistent Alterations in the Natural Killer Cell Response to Cytokines in Older Adults." *Health Psychol* 13(4) (1994): 291–8.

Glaser, R.. and J. K. Kiecolt-Glaser "Stress-induced Immune Dysfunction: Implications for Health." *Nat Rev Immunol* 5(3) (2005): 243–51.

McEwen, B. with E. N. Lasley. *The End of Stress as We Know It.* New York. Joseph Henry Press, 2002.

Sapolsky, R.M. *Why Zebras Don't Get Ulcers* 3rd ed. New York: Henry Holt, 2004.

Can Believing Make You Well?

If stress can make you sick, can believing make you well? And if we just work hard enough at it, shouldn't we just be able to think ourselves better? Logic and perhaps human nature tell us that the answers to these questions must be yes. In the 1920s the French psychoanalyst Emile Coué wrote that if one looked in the mirror every morning and recited the lines, "Day by day, in every way, I am getting better and better," one would actually get better. In the 1970s, Norman Cousins espoused laughter and positive attitude as a healing therapy. Thousands of fervent followers of these prescriptions for well-being did get better, and if their illnesses weren't resolved through these techniques alone, at least they gained the strength to fight it through. We speak of patients fighting illness, battling cancer—all terms implying active and conscious participation of the patient in the fight against disease. In fact, no physician who has dealt with dying patients would deny the power of the will to live. Fight one more month until the grandchild is born, one more week until the sister returns to say good-bye, and the patient lives; but once the will is lost, the fight is over, and the patient soon slips away.

But the question still remains: Can we consciously choose to improve our health? The answer to this question lies in knowing what portion of the systems that control our health are hardwired and unchangeable and what portions can be changed by how we think and

"Can Believing Make You Well?" Chapter 9 from *The Balance Within: The Science Connecting Health and Emotions* (Holt, 2001) by Esther M. Sternberg, M.D. Reprinted with permission.

what we believe. Believing is many things. It can be fervent prayer. It can be thoughtful meditation. It can be deep conviction. Or it can be a set of assumptions so ingrained that we don't even realize they're there. One element common to all these forms of belief is expectation—we pray, we laugh, we repeat a phrase, we take a pill, and we expect that these actions will help us heal. And at the core of such expectation is learning.

Just as we can learn a new task, we can learn to make connections between events, actions, and feelings. This form of learning, called conditioning, becomes automatic and comes from the brain's ability to associate two signals. It is the classic conditioning experiment, in which the Russian scientist Ivan Pavlov trained his dog to associate the sound of a bell with dinner so that whenever the bell would sound, the dog would salivate. A psychological stimulus is paired with a physical one, and each can then trigger a physiological response.

We all carry with us associations, some good, some bad, that have been learned through such repeated pairings. Step out of the elevator at 8 AM into a hostile workplace, and you experience all the flood of bad feelings that have battered you each day, even before your boss confronts you yet again. With such feelings come physiological responses: Your heart rate increases, you sweat, your stomach turns. If the anxiety is great enough, your blood pressure may increase—all the classic fight-or-flight physiological responses. But step out of a cold winter night into your health spa, smell a warm whiff of swimming pool chlorine, and instead your muscles relax, you feel a glow with the anticipation of the eucalyptus-scented sauna and whirlpool.

These feelings too are learned by association. We are not born with a set of beliefs that makes us respond negatively to the workplace or positively to the health spa. We learn these responses after repeated pairings of the stimuli. A workplace can elicit a positive set of physiological responses if the environment is supportive, nurturing, and rewarding instead of hostile and unsupportive. A health spa can elicit negative associations if you had an accident there, feel ashamed of your looks, or can't accomplish your goals. The common factor that can affect your health in these situations is not the physical or psychological stimulus but your body's physiological response. And such learned associations change the body's nerve and hormone responses, which ultimately affect how immune cells work. In that sense, believing can make you sick or make you well.

Perhaps if we could relearn a new set of associations, turn negative into positive, we could in some sense consciously control our health. Perhaps with practice we can learn to disconnect feelings from the events that bring them on, through conscious will, through psychotherapy, through meditation or prayer. It then takes one more step to imagine that the emotions that come attached or disconnected can trigger the nerve and hormone pathways that could change the immune system and so our physical health.

In the 1970s, and even today, the idea that the immune system could be taught was considered an outrageously heretical notion by most classical immunologists. Immune cells can't think, they can't be trained like dogs to do tricks. Immune cells respond to molecules that crash up against them, get stuck to proteins protruding on their surfaces, get gobbled up into the cell's interior, and cause other molecules to be made in the cell's protein factories and spit out—magic antibody bullets that surround the prey and destroy it. There is no room for learning here.

But in the 1970s, an American psychologist at the University of Rochester, Bob Ader, and his immunologist colleague Nick Cohen decided to test whether the immune system could be trained, like Pavlov's dog, to respond to a conditioned stimulus. They paired the sweet taste of saccharine with an anticancer drug that suppresses immune function, cyclophosphamide. They fed both the drug and the saccharine to mice over and over again. Each time the immunosuppressive drug was given, as would be expected in response to such a drug, immune cell counts went down. Then Ader and Cohen took away the drug and fed the mice saccharine alone. The immune cells fell again, this time in response to the saccharine alone. The saccharine had no intrinsic chemical ability to lower the number of immune cells—before the learning took place, it had no effect at all. The mice weren't telling their immune cells to fall, weren't thinking "Let's turn off these cells." Something automatic was happening, something that had been learned. The mice were associating the sweet taste of saccharine with the immunosuppressive drug, and after making the association, all it took was the taste of sweetness to affect the cell counts.

Ader and Cohen did this work before much was known about the molecular neurobiology of learning and before the notion was widely accepted that nerve chemicals or hormones could affect immune cell function in a physiological way. Their report in the 1980s that conditioning could actually change the immune response, and might therefore explain some part of the placebo effect, was met with derision from some scientists. Even some of the scientists who themselves were coming at the brain-immune connection from a different angle— from the stress hormone and nerve pathway route—were skeptical. I remember a conference at Copper Mountain, Colorado, where both camps met in the summer of 1987. I was there as part of Candace Pert's group. It was before I had told anyone of my findings in Lewis rats. Besedovsky and others who were just beginning to find nerve chemical connections between immune system and brain were there too. And so was Ader and his group. It had been pouring rain all week, and all fantasies of hiking in the bracing mountain air had evaporated as the drizzle and the week wore on. We were all at close quarters, and some, like me, were suffering from headaches and fatigue—the effects of the nearly 10,000 foot altitude of the place. But the discussions of science were almost continuous and intense.

In fact, although they could not yet admit it then, the work of both sides was converging and proving the same thing. Those whose studies had started at the conditioning end concluded that this part of brain function—learning—changed the way the immune cells fight disease and could maybe even partly substitute for immune active drugs. Those who started with the chemicals and hormones of the brain concluded that these compounds changed the way immune cells work and vice versa, that immune chemicals and hormones changed the way the brain responds. What was missing then to bring the two sides together was a detailed knowledge of the chemicals and nerve pathways of learning and the discovery that some of the molecules of learning are those same immune molecules, the interleukins, that make immune cells grow, divide, and mature.

What is learning if not another set of cells growing and maturing to make connections and spit out another set of chemicals in a different organ—the brain? It turns out that nerve chemicals like serotonin and immune molecules like interleukin-1 can make nerve cells grow connections. Drip a fraction of a drop of serotonin on a nerve cell in culture, and you can watch the sprouting bud through time-lapse photography through the microscope objective. At first a little hump appears, then a point, and finally an elongating filament emerges from the place on the cell membrane where the serotonin touched, as if some invisible hand has pulled it out like taffy. Does this kind of sprouting play a role in learning? Are we, as we learn, actually growing new nerve connections?

We do a task repeatedly, shakily at first: Once, twice, fifty times, and suddenly, as when we learn to ride a bicycle, play piano, or type, it clicks and the task becomes routine. Something happens to our brains and nerve cells in this process that changes them forever. On average it takes about fifty repetitions for a change to gel. And it helps to repeat the task before sleep—sleeping helps the whole thing set. There is a biological reason that your mother told you to practice piano every day, that your teacher made you write out lessons fifty times, and then to get lots of sleep besides.

It used to be thought that the adult brain did not change, that our brain cells, unlike those of children, did not grow and divide and were not malleable. But Eric Kandel, a neurobiologist at Columbia University, found otherwise. Kandel studied the lowly aplysia—a sea slug whose nervous system consists of just the simplest circuitry, and yet it learns. He discovered that nerve cells actually grow new processes, form new connections during learning. Aplysia learn in a very simple sort of way: Repeated electrical stimulation of these simple organism's nerves, the sort that occurs in higher mammals during learning tasks, produces a permanent change in the aplysia's nerve cells, a change in which new proteins are incorporated into those cells. And with these new proteins, a new cell membrane is woven that helps them bud and sprout new connections. We don't yet have proof that this same budding growth occurs in human learning, but more and more studies show that the adult human brain does change with learning. Kandel, in his lectures to students, sometimes used to bring home the point by saying that when you leave that room, if you have listened hard and learned, you will most likely leave with a few more nerve cell connections than you had before you came.

In higher order mammals there are rapidly dividing cells deep within the brain, in memory centers like the hippocampus. Such cells move up through layers of other cells to eventually settle in the calmer, more anchored areas of the brain. Such movements and cell divisions happen increasingly with learning. The newer connections that form need to be tended, fired up repeatedly until they are firm by constant repetition of a task, until this task is so deeply entrenched in memory that it becomes automatic. We don't consciously tell our brain cells to make new connections during this learning process, we don't will our cells to grow and divide, but instinctively we know what to do to keep them fired up and activated: We practice the task.

There is an element of this sort of learning in every prescription we take: We have learned that medicines can make us better. We believe it. The amount of actual improvement in illness that comes from this learned expectation is called the placebo effect. It is the psychological component of that cure. About one-third of the therapeutic effect of every pill comes from the placebo effect. Strictly defined, a placebo is any sort of "inert" treatment whose therapeutic effect is not specific for the disease or symptom it is used to treat. A sugar pill the same shape and color as a prescription drug can be used as a placebo. Today placebos are used in medical research to determine what part of a medication's effects are specific to the drug and what part of the benefit is psychological. In the first half of the twentieth century, physicians recognized that the placebo effect was a powerful healer and used placebo sugar pills to treat illness, not just to test a drug's effects. In 1946, the American physician and professor at Cornell University Eugene DuBois alluded to the power of merely receiving a prescription when he wrote:

> You cannot write a prescription without the element of placebo.
> A prayer to Jupiter starts the prescription. It carries weight, the
> weight of two or three thousand years of medicine.[1]

• • • •

Walking on the marble flagstones in the ruins of the temple to Asclepius, you feel the exhausting heat and blinding light of the full midday sun. But when Lentas was Lebena, a bustling port town in 500 B.C.E., the healers knew the power of the temple cures. It was then a quiet sanctuary far away from the city's heat and noise below. The earth was not dry and parched. A cooling spring coursed through shaded sage and mountain laurel towards the inner courtyard of the complex, just below the patients' rooms—stone chambers built into the hillside. And the now-exposed marble flagstones of the temple, hot from the sun, formed the cool marble floor of the altar's dark interior.

On arriving at the sanctuary, the ailing patient first bathed in the cooling waters of the spring, then entered the dark halls of the enclosed Asclepion and made an offering of honey cake at a small altar to the gods. Later on at night, the patient was ushered into a silent interior chamber where a priest guided him to lie down upon a pallet on the floor. There the patient slept and dreamed. Asclepius visited the patients in their dreams and, depending on the problem, tended ills with unguents and lotions and cooling fresh water, prescribed nutritious diet and exercise regimens—walking, bathing in the sea—or interpreted dreams. In the Asclepion at Corinth, patients could stroll quietly along a shaded colonnade of an inner courtyard where sunlight filtered to the center court. For the lame, a long and gently sloping ramp gave easy access to the temple and the colonnade. Adjacent to the courtyard were dining rooms where healthful food was cooked and served. Fountains and pools, couches and tables provided soothing spaces for rest and recuperation. The wealthy and the poor could participate equally since wealthy patients were expected to pay accordingly, and those who shirked were penalized.

Patients came to these sanctuaries, prayed and rested, bathed in the cleansing waters, slept and strolled, ate nutritious meals and were treated with potions and plasters and mixtures made from mountain herbs. Many were healed and left tokens of their gratitude to the healing God, anatomical votives—carved stone or clay representations of the body parts that had been healed: legs, arms, hands, fingers, genitals, breasts, heads, ears, eyes. Such body parts could be conveniently purchased, ready-made, in shops near the Asclepion. These clay statues and their accompanying inscriptions now make up an amazing inventory of testimonials to the cures of these first hospitals and health spas.

Some of the healing power of these sanctuaries could have come from the medicinal cures the priests applied. A potion called theriac, which was used from Roman times to World War II and possibly in various forms before, was concocted in the second century C.E. by Galen, the physician to the Roman emperor Marcus Aurelius. It contained many ingredients we know to be powerful drugs. Proscillaridin—a cardiac drug used widely today, comes from one of the medicinal herbs used in theriac: squill, or *Drimia maritima,* a member of the Liliaceae family. Another, rapeseed, is a source of plant estrogens, and a third constituent, frog skin, we now know contains antibiotic chemicals called maganins. Also in theriac was the seed of a species of poppy, *Papaver somniferum*—the source of opium. Similar plants containing healing chemicals were used by the ancient Greeks and when applied appropriately by a trained physician or priest could well have had medicinal healing effects. In the wrong circumstance and dose, however, they could also have harmed.

Purifying water was an essential component of all Asclepions' ritual cures, from first bath before entering the sanctuary to prescriptions for drinking from or bathing in the sacred springs. The cleanliness, cooling, and regular exercise from bathing in the sea could all have helped effect a cure. Diet and nutrition, too, were essential elements of the Asclepions' prescriptions and certainly contributed to their cures. At least some of their effect must have come from the peaceful rest away from city heat and dirt and stress. After observing the ruins of temples to Asclepius in Corinth, in Epidaurus, and at Lebena, Plutarch, writing in the first century C.E. observed:

> Why is the shrine of Asclepius outside the city? Is it that they considered it more healthful to spend their time outside the city than within its walls? In fact the Greeks, quite reasonably, have their shrines of Asclepius situated in places which are both clean and high.[2]

Some more recent historians dispute the notion that most of the beneficial effect of the Asclepions came from their health spa-like atmosphere, however, since not all Asclepions were located in such refreshing surroundings. Some lay low in swampy, mosquito-infested ground, others in heat not far from the city center. So what was the basis of the temple cures?

The temple healers flourished alongside the ancient world's burgeoning center for the scientific practice of medicine. The ancient Greek physicians, thought by some historians to be itinerant craftsmen at this time, developed skills in prognostication in order to maintain their competitive edge with clients. Through thoughtful listening to patients' complaints and careful observations of patients' physical signs, these physician-craftsmen noticed patterns of disease that could be used to predict its course. And since the best prognosticators attracted the most clients, the more sensitive the inventory of signs and symptoms that could be compiled, the more successful the physician. From such practical beginnings, these Greek physicians' approach became the foundation upon which modern medical diagnosis is based. A patient's history and a physical exam, when performed thoroughly, are still a physician's most powerful diagnostic and prognostic tools.

The major ingredient that set apart temple healers from these practical physicians and their developing science was patients' beliefs that prayer and the gods would heal. The other components of the cures—diet, a balance of exercise and rest, herbal cures—were all also practiced by physicians or craftsmen of the day, not gods but mortals like Hippocrates. It was fervent prayer and expectation that brought the sick to these shrines, often with the blessing of their physicians who, when mortal cures had failed, recognized the immense power of prayer. It must have been the power of belief that forged the temple cures: the ultimate placebo. To say this is not to denigrate their effect: The placebo is a very potent cure, since at least one-third of the effect of any cure, whether modern medication or a health regimen of any sort, comes from the belief that it will cure—from the placebo effect.

• • • •

The separation between scientific medicine and the parallel practice of priestly cures began with the cult of Asclepius and continued through early Christian times up through the Renaissance and, with an ever-widening gulf, to our modern day. In Padua, the University of Padua's botanical garden is steps across the cobblestone square from the San Antonio Cathedral, named for the patron saint of healing. The university's anatomical dissecting theater is a few short blocks away. While Renaissance scientists classified and planted medicinal herbs in that garden and defined anatomy in the dissecting theater, pilgrims came in droves to the cathedral to pray to St. Anthony. Great Renaissance artists and sculptors adorned his shrine. The healed left tokens of their gratitude, small silver hearts and limbs in thanks—echoes of the anatomical votives left by ancient Greeks to Asclepius.

In nineteenth century Lourdes, miracle cures were effected by those who saw the Virgin Mary come to them as if in a dream. And in Montreal, at the turn of the twentieth century, a great gray limestone and now weathered green copper-domed shrine, St. Joseph's Oratory, was built to Brother André, a humble priest who cured with the laying on of hands. The sick still labor up hundreds of stone steps to reach the shrine, on the northwestern slopes of Mount Royal, to enter and pray. They leave their crutches behind as testimonials to the healing power of their saint: more echoes of the votives of the past.

Scientists cannot explain these cures, and with a failure to understand often comes skepticism and scorn. But if belief in the power of a drug to cure gives it at least a third of its ability to heal, why shouldn't prayer and fervent belief alone be an effective cure, which works in part through those same nerve pathways and hormones that transduce the placebo effect?

There are two sides to prayer—one is what happens to the believer praying, and the other is the prayer itself. Science can neither presume to have an explanation nor refute or support the intrinsic power of a prayer. But we can now address the first part of the equation—the matters that change in the person praying. If prayers do heal, and they surely do, at least a part of their effect must be placebo: the belief that they will heal. To say that part of healing brought on by the act of praying could come via the placebo effect is not to say it is fake, but rather to give it a very real explanation. However the placebo effect is brought into action, whether by making a prayer or believing in a pill, once in play it acts through well-defined nerve pathways and molecules—molecules that can have profound effects on how immune cells function. A part of prayer's effect therefore might come from removing stress—reversing that burst of hormones that can suppress immune cell function. Another part of that effect might come from beneficial nerve chemicals that actively counteract the stress response.

Recall the ways that novelty brings stress—through loss of something old and anxiety over unfamiliar newness. As newness fades, so too does stress and all the hormone bursts that can exacerbate illness. One way we soothe the stress of change and loss is with old, familiar ritual. There is a ritual in building a fire in a hearth, a ritual that carries with it its own warm and soothing space, even amid the tumult of the unfamiliar. The systematic actions of piling logs on kindling, the smells of burning wood, the mesmerizing flames, the warmth are all familiar and bring a sense of peace. All these sensory inputs: the flickering light, the hickory smoke, the cold outdoors and crunchy snow may hearken back to childhood holidays and to a simpler time of safety and less responsibility. If we focus on the fire, we can block out the now-threatening world around us.

But soothing rituals needn't only re-create the physical. We can re-create a soothing familiar space in our mind through thought and words and song. These rituals are even more portable than actions like building a fire. These are the rituals of prayer. We can carry them within us and pull them out at any time and any place—at work, at home, in a house of God. We need just close our eyes and we are there, back in that old familiar soothing place that banishes anxiety and grief and sadness with familiarity.

At least one element of prayer that helps remove stress and helps achieve a sense of peace is the repeated performance of a set of actions until they become automatic. In the automaticity of ritual, a kind of familiarity is reached through learning. It is as if the ritual is the door through which the believer leaves the hurly-burly world behind and steps into a calming space. Our need for such escapes is present all our lives and reflected in the stories we grew up on. The magic talismans of children's literature all help in these escapes: Slip on the magic rings in C. S. Lewis's *The Lion, The Witch and the Wardrobe*, and you can jump into the dark magic pools in the wood between the worlds and enter new worlds. But lose the ring, and instead you land in mud. At times of stress and turmoil, there is a longing of the human spirit to step like magic into such pools or through such doors, into a child's world of nurturance and peace.

In fact, often the believer does step into a familiar physical space. The ancient Greeks stepped into their temples; later, Christians walked into awe-inspiring Gothic cathedrals; modern worshippers go to the temples, churches, and mosques of their own particular faiths. In all this, the worshipper leaves both an over-stimulating and often unfamiliar physical and mental world for a time to step into a calming, familiar place of prayer—wherever that may be. Because even if the worshipper is in novel surroundings—the person who has moved homes, is in a new city, is in a new psychological place of divorce or grieving—there is a constancy to temple, church or mosque and a constancy to ritual and prayer that gives familiarity. With familiarity comes resolution of anxiety. And with familiarity also comes a lowering of stress hormones that peaked during novelty. So it may be that familiarity of ritual and of prayer affords the same dampening of stress response and anxiety as does learning familiarity with a novel space. If that's the case, then soothing prayer may soothe immune responses too—remove them from the vicelike grip of steroid hormones that suppress their function.

Indeed, although the mechanisms still need to be proven, researchers like Harold Koenig of Duke University are now finding in large epidemiological studies (close to one thousand people) that religious observance is associated with less medical illness and lower rates of hospital admissions. On a smaller scale, for over a decade AIDS researchers have shown an effect of belief and expectations on course and outcome of disease. Several other researchers have conducted studies with AIDS and HIV-positive patients and found similar results. Neil Schneiderman, a psychologist at the University of Miami in Coral Gables, Florida, found that stress management training in HIV-positive men buffered not only their feelings of stress but also their cortisol and other stress hormone responses. Margaret Kemeny and her group at the University of California in Los Angeles studied coping patterns in bereaved HIV-positive men. They found that those who processed their loss and found meaning in it had less rapid decreases in number of helper or CD-4–type lymphocytes (those lymphocytes that rapidly fall with progression of AIDS) and lower death rates from AIDS than men who didn't have such positive response patterns to stressful events. This same group studied non-AIDS subjects and also found an association between mood, expectancy, and immune cell responses. The more optimistic the persons, the less they perceived an event as stressful, the more robust were their immune cell responses.

Putting all these studies together with what we know of the suppressive effects of stress hormones on immune responses, one could infer that the healing effect of belief and expectation might come only through removal of stress and reduction of the immune-suppressing hormonal burst. But could there also be a positive effect of prayer—one in which the addition of other soothing molecules plays a role in healing as much as the subtraction of stressful ones? Herbert Benson, a professor of psychiatry at Harvard University School of Medicine, has proposed that there is indeed such a positive response that can be brought into play by all sorts of soothing actions, including prayer and meditation. This "relaxation response" is a stereotypical physiological response made up of a cascade of nerve chemicals and hormones, a sort of mirror-image of Selye's stress response.

• • • •

Across Mount Royal from St. Joseph's Oratory, a pleasant walk through landscaped park and past some wilder woods, is McGill University's medical school building. A round cylinder of glass and steel, the building perches on the southeastern face of the largest of Mount Royal's several extinct volcanic domes, overlooking Montreal's downtown skyline and the St. Lawrence river. In the 1970s, in his introductory psychology class to the medical students, Ron Melzack, a psychologist and expert in pain pathways, described injured soldiers at the Anzio Beachhead in World War II. These men, pulled from the carnage, severely injured, missing limbs, nonetheless felt no pain. For them the war was over. They were going home. Loss of limb meant they were saved, and somehow this strong positive psychological meaning of the event overrode the physical component of the pain.

When a limb is cut, electrical signals race from tiny nerve endings in the skin and muscle up through those nerve trunks the anatomists discovered, back to the spinal cord. There they enter the spinal cord at bulbous switching stations, tangles of nerve processes closely apposed on nerve cell bodies whose long processes cross the spinal cord to their cable paths on the opposite side. From here these wirelike nerve bundles thread up the spinal cord to another switching station at the base of the brain, and from there another relay set of nerve fibers leads into an area of brain just above the hypothalamus called the thalamus. This structure deep within the brain shows the same geographical somatotropic distribution of nerve cells as the sensory map that Penfield and Milner described. In this way, when the skin is cut you immediately know where that cut is on the body, and you feel pain. All this happens in a fraction of a second.

But there are also descending nerve pathways, cable paths in which electrical signals move downward through the spinal cord. The source of electrical spikes that move along these trunks are the parts of the brain that govern thought and those amorphous parts that we are just beginning to understand, the centers for emotion. These centers and the signals that they send can block pain signals that arise at sites of injury and then move up the spinal cord. So, the circuitry of pain includes not only a sensory element but wiring that can dampen pain through psychological tinge.

The pain of childbirth is said to be one of the ten worst pains in medicine. And yet, a woman can be taught in part to control that pain. The pain is there; it doesn't go away. But one can be distracted from it by rhythmic breathing and concentration. At least as important as the mantras and rituals learned in birthing classes is the soothing presence of a guiding nurse or spouse. This psychological support numbs the component of the pain that comes from fear. No matter how knowledgeable the mother is about anatomy and the physiological process of childbirth, at the moment of an intense contraction, sheer

terror takes over besides the pain. Because the sensations are so un-
natural, so never felt before, that is, to your conscious brain, it feels as
if your insides are being ripped out. Knowing this is not the case, being
reminded of it by a trusted presence, dissipates the fearful part of pain.
Learning and association—conditioning—in this setting can help
relieve some pain.

The way this is achieved is through a complex wiring system of
nerves connecting the brain's higher centers to the spinal cord. It is
here that these nerves meet other nerves that send pain signals from
the limbs and organs down below. If you crack the spinal column,
there between its hard bony arches and the vertebral column's thick
supporting cylinders of bone lies the glistening spinal cord. Cut hori-
zontally through the spinal cord, and you see a butterfly-like imprint:
a gray center surrounded by a white outer layer. The soft gray spongy
part is where the nerve cell bodies lie, and in the whiter areas are the
cable trunks—the wirelike fibers of each nerve. The butterfly's horn-
shaped parts, called dorsal horns because of their shape and the back
(or dorsal) part of the column where they lie, form a kind of railroad
switching yard where tracks from many parts converge. Here the long
nerves running up from skin and muscle meet with other long nerves
running on to the brain. Shorter nerves, so short that their fibers don't
extend outside the dorsal horns, act like switches on the railroad track—
switches that can shut off one track and activate another.

Electrical impulses from the higher learning centers travel down
the spinal cord and end on other nerves whose Morse code of electrical discharges, moving up the spinal cord, would signal pain. These
downward signals can shift the track and thus block pain. But switches
in the spinal cord are not mechanical—the nervous system relies on
chemicals, called neuropeptides or neurotransmitters, to do the job.
These chemicals, released from nerves whose electrical signals are head-
ing down descending pain pathways, or those released from the short
inhibitory neurons in the dorsal horns, can dampen pain and block
incoming pain signals by temporarily paralyzing the electrical activity of target cells. Among the chemicals that can do this are the endogenous opiates, or endorphins.

• • • •

If you face the sea from the hill on which the temple to Asclepius
stands in Lentas, you look south over the shining Mediterranean to-

wards Egypt. But if you turn and face the north, you will look out over the fertile valley that fills the center of the island. On the other side of this valley lie the ruins of the most powerful city of the Minoan civilization, which flourished around 1900–1500 B.C.E. It is the palace of Knossos—home of King Minos and the myth of the Minotaur. Among the ruins found in Knossos, dating from about 3500 B.C.E., is a terra-cotta head—an image of a sleeping goddess with a beatific smile and closed eyes. On her head is a crown of three slit poppy pods.

There is little doubt that the opium poppy was used—indeed cultivated—by the ancients who inhabited the Mediterranean basin. It is equally clear that these civilizations knew of its medicinal and altering effects. Even the Sumerians, who inhabited Mesopotamia in 3400 B.C.E., used two written symbols for the poppy: "joy plant."

If, after it has bloomed, you slit the ripe pod of the opium poppy with a sharp knife, a white sap oozes from it. It looks as if someone has tried to repair the pod with too much children's school glue. In the sun, the sap dries down to a black gum containing a mixture of chemicals that can induce a trancelike sleep and silence pain. Multiringed structures made up of carbon and hydrogen atoms, these chemicals are called opiate alkaloids and include codeine and morphine. Extracted, purified, and synthesized, many of them are used in medicine today for pain and sedation. And they are, and have been for centuries, drugs of abuse.

The reason these drugs work is that they mimic molecules made by nerve cells, the neuropeptides and neurotransmitters. Each different opiate molecule fits neatly into a protein seat that protrudes from the nerve cells' surface. Once the drug has settled in its cove, it trips another protein latched onto the receptor's root, dangling inside the cell. This then triggers a cascade of protein shifts that lead to changes in the cell's electrical activity. The opiate drugs work because their three-dimensional shape is identical to the shape of parts of the endorphins, which are meant to lock into these receptors. So, while we tend to think only of external drugs as having real painkilling power, the body's own endorphins can shut down pain just as easily and well as morphine.

Opiates produce their effects on pain in many ways. When released from nerves within the dorsal horns, they can block the electrical activity of pain nerve fibers sending signals up the spinal cord. When released from higher centers, they can increase the firing rate of nerve fibers whose electrical spikes run down the spinal cord, and thus they can block the upward traffic. In a center at the base of the brain, just above where the spinal cord widens to a stem, in an area called the brain stem, there are two kinds of cells called "on" and "off" cells. These cells can switch on pain paths, or they can switch them off. Morphine and other opiates also make off cells work harder. (The antimorphine drug naloxone turns "on" cells on and "off" cells off.) Even higher brain centers can also be shut down by opiate drugs and endogenous endorphins. These include the hypothalamus, the amygdala, and higher regions that govern thought. It is by blocking nerve cells in these parts of brain that opiates cloud thinking, dull anxiety, and also dull pain.

Where do the endogenous opiates come from? They come from nerve cells in many parts of the brain. These cells produce the molecules that soothe us, such as the enkephalins, short strings of amino acids with opiate-like effects. In a sort of perfect symmetry, they are made and squirted out by the same cells in the hypothalamus that make the stress hormone CRH. Other opiate peptides are made in cells within the brain stem and spinal cord. The same kinds of things that make the hypothalamic cells release their stress hormones also make them release these numbing, lulling molecules. It is as if by grand design that the molecules that oppose stress are there to keep the whole in balance. It is not hard to imagine, then, how such nerve circuits and neurotransmitters can explain the effects of placebo on pain. And if such learning and expectation are part of what we call belief, why could not believing change our sense of pain? And if this is the case, why couldn't learned and conditioned beliefs also change the course of inflammation through the same molecules and nerve routes? Indeed, it turns out that blocking the body's own opiate molecules with drugs can block those immune-suppressive effects of conditioning that Bob Ader showed in mice.

Surgically blocking spinal pain pathways can also change the course of inflammation. Two rheumatologists from California, Jon Levine and Paul Green, took advantage of the body's symmetry in nerves and joints and did just that. They cut the nerves on one side in rats, then treated the animals with an oil that caused arthritis. While arthritis developed in the joints on the side where the spinal cord had not been touched, none developed on the side that had been cut. This fit with clinical observations in people who had suffered a paralyzing stroke. If arthritis develops in such a patient, it affects only the joints on the side that is not paralyzed. So these patients and what happened to the rats tell us that something in the nerve pathways in the spinal cord allows arthritis to develop, and blocking these routes stops arthritis in its track. That something could very well be the very molecules released by nerves springing from the spinal cord and feeding those areas of inflammation in the joints and tissues.

• • • •

When you bite into a hot chili pepper or a Hungarian red pepper, you first feel a sting and then a burning in your tongue. This is because a substance in the pepper called capsaicin is binding to receptors on pain fibers in the tongue. The capsaicin makes these nerve fibers release their contained neurotransmitter, a short protein or peptide called Substance P. So the sting you feel and then the burning comes from pain signals transmitted through these very rapid firing nerves. As you eat more hot chili peppers, some of these nerve fibers die back, and so the more you eat, the more you need to eat in order to feel the zing.

Substance P-containing nerve fibers form a rich and lacey lattice work in skin and joints. Where they are particularly dense, pain is most sensitively felt. During inflammation, the surrounding irritation can cause these nerves to empty their packets of Substance P into the inflammatory site—the joint space, for instance, in arthritis. And when this happens, Substance P itself makes inflammation worse. Because, it turns out, Substance P attracts and then turns on immune cells.

In the 1980s and 1990s, immunologists like Ed Goetzl, Don Payan, and Jon Levine in California and Andres Stanisz and Joel Weinstock in Canada decided to test the effects of Substance P on immune cells grown in tissue culture and measure it at sites of inflammation. They did this because when Substance P, and peptides like it, are injected into skin, a wheal and flare develop—a hive, just like what allergic people get when they touch or eat the thing that makes them allergic.

These scientists wondered whether Substance P could activate macrophages, those garbage collector cells that gobble debris. Payan and Goetzl added Substance P to macrophages and found that the cells gobbled more. The cells had become activated, and when activated they started spewing out their own transmitter molecules, those chemical protein signals called cytokines. They made interleukin-1, and this in turn made lymphocytes make interleukin-2. Others later searched for and found Substance P in inflammatory cells and nerves at sites of inflammation. And so, a neuropeptide that in the nervous system communicates pain, at sites of inflammation was calling in and activating immune cells and amplifying inflammation. This sequence fits with what we know of injury: An inflamed site hurts where it looks inflamed. It goes back to the old Latin description of the signs of inflammation: dolor, rubor, calor, turgor—pain, redness, heat and swelling. All these signs come from the effects of those nerve chemicals and immune molecules spewing out in inflamed tissue.

At the same time, John Bienenstock, an immunologist, was studying mast cells in Hamilton, a small university town in the western part of Canada's province of Ontario. Mast cells are a type of white blood cell that release a chemical called histamine during an allergic reaction. Anyone who has had an allergic reaction will know what histamine is and how it makes you feel. It is the chemical that causes skin to swell up and become itchy when you get a hive. It is the chemical that makes you sneeze and makes your nose run and eyes water when you inhale pollen or dust. And it is the chemical whose action is blocked by those pills that you can buy in any grocery store for allergy symptoms—antihistamines. It is released from small sacs contained in mast cells—sacs that when stained with the right dye look like blue polka dots inside these cells. When an allergic person comes into contact with an allergen—a protein or chemical that causes allergies—the mast cells' histamine-containing sacs empty. It is the released histamine that triggers the itching, redness and swelling of allergic reaction.

Bienenstock wondered whether the itching results from irritation of nerve endings. He began to observe mast cells in tissues and noticed that they accumulate around nerve endings of nerves that contain the nerve chemical serotonin. Bienenstock began to do time-lapse photography of these nerve endings. Under the microscope lens of the time-lapse camera, he could watch the mast cells crawl along nerve endings and attach themselves closely to the nerve fibers—like barnacles on a rope. Even under an electron microscope, the connection between mast cells and nerve endings bore a striking resemblance to connections between nerve endings themselves—the synapses. These synapses are the tiny gulfs of fluid between cells across which information, transmitted as electrical charges along nerves, must jump. But the electrical charge can't jump across the space, and so, instead, when the charge reaches the end of the nerve, it empties tiny sacs of chemicals, the neurotransmitters, into the watery space. These neurotransmitters spread across the space to the opposite shore, where another charge is triggered to go racing down the next nerve until the sequence in the circuit is complete.

What John Bienenstock observed by time-lapse photography is that the mast cells moved so close to nerve endings that they formed connections that looked like synapses. Why couldn't these immune cells be communicating with the nerves against which they nuzzled by emptying the contents of their sacs into the fluid space between? So it appeared that this was yet another way in which immune system and nervous system communicated and yet another way in which the nervous system might regulate disease. Bienenstock's findings also suggested a way that serotonin released from nerves might act in natural settings to activate immune cells in the body, not just in the tissue culture dish.

The striking thing about all these effects of nerve chemicals is that most seem to activate immune cells and so increase inflammation. There is one group of nerve chemicals, however, that when added directly to immune cells turns down their activity and could directly shut off inflammation. These are the opiates. Whether drugs or endogenously manufactured proteins, the opiate morphine, endorphins, and enkephalins all dampen the ability of immune cells to fight infection. The way these compounds exert their effects is by first binding to receptors on the surface of immune cells. So here's another symmetry of nature, another level at which these two great systems communicate: Receptors for nerve chemicals are found on immune cells, and nerve chemicals change the way immune cells function.

Since so many different chemicals that come through nerves coursing down the spinal cord from the brain can change the way immune cells work—tune them up or tune them down—it is logical to expect that changing the flow of such nerve chemicals by any mechanism could alter inflammation. So, if interfering with the flow with surgical cuts or drug treatment can block arthritis, why couldn't conditioning and belief do so as well? The missing link to complete this circle is an understanding of what controls the hormones and nerve chemicals of our brain's stress and relaxation pathways. If learning, conditioning, ritual, prayer, and meditation downshift the stress response, decrease stress hormones, and allow enkephalins, endorphins, and other molecules to play a greater role, then such molecules might shift the balance too of nerve chemicals flowing down the spinal cord from those that induce pain and inflammation to those that tone it down. Although this has not yet been proved, it just remains for this old-new science to systematically define the paths by which thoughts and beliefs formed by learning and association in the cortex of the brain could send signals down through spinal cord and nerves to change immune cell function and disease at sites of inflammation.

NOTES

[1] Eugene F. Dubois, "The Use of Placebos in Therapy," Cornell Conferences on Therapy, 1946.

[2] Plutarchus, "Aetia Romana," in *Asclepius: Collection and Interpretation of the Testimonies*, E.J. Edelstein and L. Edelstein (Baltimore: Johns Hopkins Univ. Press, 1945).

6

The Neural Bases of Placebo
Effects in Pain

LAUREN Y. ATLAS
AND TOR D. WAGER

Introduction

Placebo effects have a rich and controversial history and have been the focus of intrigue and heated debate throughout the past century. Their role in the healing professions is so significant that several researchers have written, "The history of medicine [is the] history of the placebo effect" (de la Fuente-Fernandez, Schulzer, and Stoessl 2004; Kradin 2004; A. K. Shapiro and Morris 1978). Some have argued that medical practitioners should be encouraged and even trained to take advantage of the healing power of placebos in their practices, while others have argued that clinical placebo administration is deceptive and unethical. Even the existence of placebo effects has been challenged; opponents have asserted that placebo administration is akin to quackery and that placebo responders are malingerers without real diseases. By contrast, the strongest proponents of placebo research have asserted that understanding the mechanisms of the placebo response will give us more insight into "self-healing competencies" (Hall, Dugan, Zheng, and Mishra 2001).

This controversy stems from several sources. First, early researchers did not and could not, using the tools available at the time—investigate the neurobiological mechanisms of placebo effects. The lack of plausible mechanisms made it difficult to agree on what counts as a placebo effect and to systematically consider different sources of placebo responses in different disease states and outcome measures. Second, many clinical studies were not designed to assess the strength and causes of placebo effects, and so placebo effects in many of these studies are confounded with statistical biases and potential artifacts related to study sampling and the natural course of disease. Finally, findings of placebo effects in many studies are based purely on self-reported improvements, which, skeptics are quick to point out, might be caused by cognitive and social biases unrelated to the clinical course of disease.

In recent years, a resurgence of experimental research designed specifically to study the effects of placebo treatments has shed considerable light on the potential mechanisms of placebo responses, providing a new look at whether, and under what conditions, thought patterns such as expectation, motivation, and belief affect health. These studies have used pharmacological manipulations and new techniques for recording activity in the functioning human brain, including event-related electrical potentials (ERPs), magnetic potentials using magnetoencephalography (MEG), intra-cranial electrical recording in humans, functional magnetic resonance imaging (fMRI), and positron emission tomography (PET). Together, these techniques are beginning to piece together the electrical and neurochemical pathways in the brain that can, under certain circumstances, shape perceptual, emotional, and physiological aspects of pain and other disorders.

The emerging picture painted by these techniques is that placebo treatments work by eliciting a combination of positive expectations and specific learning in the brain circuitry, which connects the frontal cortex with lower-level brain stem centers that regulate physiological responses in the body. Neurochemically, opioids and dopamine are two chemical messenger systems that have been implicated in these recent studies. Both neurochemical systems appear to be principal players in positive emotion and motivation. Thus, the effects of placebo treatments may share much in common with the widely-studied effects of emotion and stress on health. This emerging view is corroborated by the fact that the three clinical domains in which evidence of placebo effects is most convincing—pain, Parkinson's disease, and depression—all appear to share common neurocircuitry in the emotional and motivational centers of the brain.

Placebo treatments, placebo effects, and placebo responses

A *placebo treatment* is one that is expected to have no direct physical or pharmacological benefit—for example, a starch capsule given for anxiety or pain, or a surgery where the critical surgical procedure is not performed. For this reason, placebos are routinely used as control or baseline conditions in clinical studies. The effects of therapeutic treatments are compared with placebo treatment, controlling for "nonspecific" aspects of the treatment, including effects of participating in the study and other effects discussed below. However, placebo treatments have also frequently been used to actually treat a variety of ailments; they have had a place in the healer's repertoire for thousands of years (A. K. Shapiro and E. Shapiro 1999) and are used as clinical treatments by physicians in industrialized countries today with surprising frequency (Sherman and Hickner 2008).

The mere fact that a patient improves on a clinical outcome measure after a placebo treatment does not prove the power of the placebo; this complexity is one important source of the controversy mentioned earlier. After all, the patient might have improved spontaneously or due to some factor (perhaps a change of diet or exercise) other than the placebo treatment itself. For example, a patient might report reduced knee pain after a sham surgery (Moseley, Wray, Kuykendall, Willis, and Landon 1996), but this does not definitively prove that the placebo surgery was responsible for the reduction. The patient may have been on the mend anyway. What one would like to know is whether the placebo *caused* the reduction in pain. For that, one would have to know what *would have happened* had the same patient not received the placebo treatment.

While one can never know what would have happened in any particular instance if things had been done differently, researchers have developed some ways of probing the fundamentally unobservable difference between two different courses of action. Patients are assigned to different treatments—in our knee example, placebo treatment and no treatment—at random. If assignment is random and the sample is large enough, the researcher might reasonably assume that the two groups are the same in all other ways besides the type of treatment given. By comparing the placebo group with the no-treatment (or natural history) group, one can assess the effect of placebo treatment and control for factors associated with the natural course of disease.

Improvements observed in the placebo group above and beyond those observed in the no-treatment group are referred to as *placebo effects.* Thus, not all improvements on placebo treatments count as placebo effects. To unequivocally demonstrate a placebo effect, one must perform a controlled study comparing a placebo treatment to a natural history control group.

To the degree that placebo treatments are healing agents, their power lies in the psychobiological context surrounding treatment (Moerman and Jonas 2002), resulting in an active response in the brain and body of the patient. Placebo treatments, by definition, are sensory cues (visual stimuli, sounds, touch, taste, odors, or combinations of these) that impact the brain but do not specifically affect health-related outcomes (e.g., reported pain, activity in relevant brain areas, clinical symptomatology) by more direct means. Thus, for a placebo to have an actual effect, it must induce some active response in the brain that causes a therapeutic change in behavior, experience, or physiology that in turn influences the outcome. We refer to the active process of perceiving and interpreting these sensory cues as a *placebo response.*

Do placebo effects exist?

The ultimate question with regard to placebo, put forth by Wilkins (Wilkins 1985), is "Which activities, delivered by which therapists in which settings, to which patients receiving which placebos, cause improvement for which complaints?"

On the one hand, placebo effects appear to be endemic across a wide variety of disease conditions and placebo treatments. Improvements after placebo treatments have been reported in a wide variety of disorders, ranging from pain to hypertension to mortality. However, as we argue above, improvements on placebo treatment do not necessarily entail active placebo responses. Without a placebo response, there can be no placebo effects—that is, no causal effects of placebo treatment. Kienle and Kiene (1997) reviewed evidence for clinical placebo effects and found that in many cases effects attributed to placebo treatment could be explained in other ways (as a byproduct of missing or improper experimental controls, sampling bias, and other factors). In fact, they identified twenty-one different kinds of methodological issues with these studies that could lead to apparent placebo effects.

More recently, Hrobjartsson and Gotzsche (2001, 2004) have taken a stronger stance. They conducted two meta-analyses of clinical placebo effects across a range of conditions, including pain, obesity, asthma, hypertension, insomnia, anxiety, and others. While a key component of Kienle and Kiene's criticism of reported placebo effects was the lack of adequate controls in studies that purported to show placebo effects, Hrobjartsson and Gotszche took care to identify clinical studies that contained no-treatment control groups against which to evaluate the effects of placebo treatment.

In the first study, they examined evidence for placebo effects in 114 studies. The main analyses grouped different disorders together (which has subsequently been criticized (I. Kirsch and Scoboria 2001)). They examined both binary outcomes, such as the number of smokers vs. nonsmokers in placebo and no-treatment groups, and continuous outcomes, such as the number of cigarettes smoked. Overall, binary outcomes across the 114 trials showed no overall benefit of placebo, though continuous outcomes showed a significant benefit with placebo. Though the authors were more interested in binary outcomes, perhaps because binary classifications are often used to categorize patient groups and quantify recovery, continuous outcomes provide a more sensitive measure because most health-related outcomes follow continuous distributions.

For example, individuals have a range of blood pressure levels on a continuous scale, and there is no magic cutoff point at which the risk of heart attack or stroke suddenly jumps up; however, for clinical purposes, individuals are classified as having high blood pressure if their blood pressure exceeds a fixed cutoff value. Thus, a world-class sprinter with blood pressure on the low end of normal and an overweight lawyer with blood pressure just under the cutoff would both be classified as "normal," though the actual blood pressure values certainly contain information about health risks.

Although the authors of these meta-analyses focused on the lack of placebo effects in binary outcomes, it is interesting to note that placebo effect sizes in several areas were relatively large, though they did not reach statistical significance. These effect sizes are shown in Table 1. As the table shows, the most widely studied condition was physical pain, with 1,602 patients in twenty-seven separate studies. Pain shows a large and significant effect size, with a Cohen's d value (the mean placebo effect divided by its standard deviation) of 0.27.

Although the effect sizes in every other condition besides insomnia and anxiety were actually larger than that for pain, pain was found to be the only condition in which placebos were systematically found to have therapeutic effects. The authors focused on the subjective nature of the pain reporting process and suggested that placebo effects were artifacts of demand characteristics and reporting biases rather than powerful therapeutic phenomena.

Table 1. Meta-analysis results						
Disorder	N	Studies	Cohen's d	Confidence Interval		
Pain	1602	27	0.27	(0.40	to	0.15)
Obesity	128	5	0.40	(0.92	to	0.12)
Asthma	81	3	0.34	(0.83	to	0.14)
Hypertension	129	7	0.32	(0.78	to	0.13)
Insomnia	100	5	0.26	(0.66	to	0.13)
Anxiety	257	6	0.06	(0.31	to	0.18)
Note: Adapted from Hrobjartsson and Gotzsche 2001						

Another interesting finding from the meta-analysis is that there was evidence for significant heterogeneity across the studies, indicating that placebo effects may have been prominent in some studies and not others. Part of this heterogeneity surely relates to the many illnesses that were lumped together in the analyses. Another part relates perhaps to factors that are harder to quantify and are not described in research reports, such as the caring qualities and presence of the human research staff.

A subsequent meta-analysis (Meissner, Distel, and Mitzdorf 2007) analyzed many of the same studies and came to somewhat different conclusions. They first collected a group of thirty-four placebo-controlled clinical studies culled from the huge clinical trial literature. Studies of clinical conditions that were stable over time were selected, whether or not they included no-treatment control groups. An exploratory analysis identified two kinds of clinical outcomes: physical and biochemical. Physical outcomes, such as hypertension and airway responsivity in asthma, showed evidence for improvement with placebo treatment during the course of the study, suggesting that placebo effects may exist in these outcome measures. Biochemical outcomes, including measures related to heart failure, infection, cholesterol, and rheumatoid arthritis, showed virtually no evidence for improvement on placebo treatment.

These groupings were applied to a second set of studies identified because they included no-treatment control groups, and thus the effects of placebo treatment itself could be more directly addressed. Analysis of this second data set confirmed that placebo effects in physical outcomes, but not biochemical outcomes, could be reliably identified. These results point out two important aspects of placebo responses: First, in contrast to the assertions of Hrobjartsson and Gotzsche, this meta-analysis of adequately controlled clinical trials does indeed offer evidence of systematic placebo effects in nonsubjective outcomes. Second, this study points to the necessity of investigating the *mechanisms* of placebo responses to get a better handle on why placebo effects are more consistently seen in physical, but not biochemical, outcomes.

Although Hrobjartsson and Gotzsche were right to be skeptical of the range of effects that have been called placebo effects, neither of these clinical meta-analyses include experimental studies designed specifically to address placebo effects and their mechanisms. Experimental studies involve control conditions that rule out virtually all the problematic artifacts discussed by Kienle and Kiene (1997) and typically involve stronger manipulation of expectancies than the typical double-blind conditions in clinical trials, in which patients are told that they may receive either active treatment or placebo. Patients taking part in clinical trials may guess at which treatment they received, and they may thus develop idiosyncratic expectations. Some patients receiving placebo believe they're receiving an active drug, but many are likely to believe they're receiving the placebo treatment, weakening the placebo response.

For this reason, studies that manipulate expectations experimentally (telling all participants that a placebo is an effective treatment and comparing this to a control substance that is said to have no effect) produce stronger placebo effects than double-blind clinical trials (Vase, Riley, and Price 2002). Likewise, improvement in depression is stronger in drug comparison studies, in which patients know they will get an active drug, than in double-blind studies (Rutherford, Sneed, and Roose submitted). Thus, double-blind studies provide relatively weak expectancies of improvement and thus relatively weak placebo responses.

Controlled experimental studies have found evidence for placebo effects (and thus evidence for active placebo responses) in a wide variety of conditions, including reported pain (Benedetti 2007; Benedetti and Amanzio 1997; De Pascalis, Chiaradia, and Carotenuto 2002; Harrington 1999; Liberman 1964; Montgomery and Kirsch 1997; Price et al. 1999; Vase, Robinson, Verne, and Price 2005; N. J. Voudouris, Peck, and Coleman 1985; Wager, Matre, and Casey 2006; Wager et al. 2004; Wager, Scott, and Zubieta 2007), asthma (Kemeny et al. 2007), cortisol release (Benedetti, Amanzio, Vighetti, and Asteggiano 2006; Benedetti et al. 2003; Johansen, Brox, and Flaten 2003), depression (Mayberg et al. 2002), Parkinson's disease (Benedetti et al. 2004; Colloca, Lopiano, Lanotte, and Benedetti 2004; de la Fuente-Fernandez et al. 2001; Pollo et al. 2002), conditioned immunosuppression (Goebel et al. 2002), allergic rhinitis (Goebel, Meykadeh, Kou, Schedlowski, and Hengge in press), negative emotion (Petrovic et al. 2005), insomnia (Storms and Nisbett 1970), respiratory function (Benedetti et al. 1998; Benedetti, Amanzio, Baldi, Casadio, and Maggi 1999) and cardiovascular function (Lanotte et al. 2005; Pollo, Vighetti, Rainero, and Benedetti 2003).

As with the clinical studies, the most commonly reported effect is in pain, and pain has been most intensively studied. Pain is in many ways an ideal model system for studying placebo effects because it is clinically relevant, but it can also be applied experimentally and studied quantitatively in the laboratory. In addition, much is known about the neurobiology of pain that can provide insight into the mechanisms by which it works, in particular the brain-body pathways that participate in the creation of the pain experience and its effects on the body. This in turn allows us to use pain as a model system in which to investigate the mechanisms by which placebo responses modulate perception and physiology.

Indeed, the lack of plausible identifiable mechanisms for placebo responses may be at the root of the controversy surrounding their existence. Understanding the mechanisms of placebo responses across various disorders and in placebo analgesia as a model system can provide some guiding principles that shed light on the complex question of "Which activities . . . in which settings . . . to which patients . . .

cause improvement for which complaints." Brain imaging and related studies are beginning to address the question of which brain systems participate in placebo analgesia (Benedetti et al. 1998; Benedetti, Amanzio, and Maggi 1995; Benedetti et al. 2006; Benedetti, Lanotte, Lopiano, and Colloca 2007; Bingel, Lorenz, Schoell, Weiller, and Buchel 2006; Petrovic, Kalso, Petersson, and Ingvar 2002; Price, Craggs, Verne, Perlstein, and Robinson 2007; Scott et al. 2007, 2008; Wager et al. 2006; Wager et al. 2004; Wager et al. 2007; Zubieta et al. 2005; Zubieta, Yau, Scott, and Stohler 2006). We turn in the following sections to a more detailed investigation of laboratory placebo analgesia studies and some of these new findings.

The laboratory placebo experiment

In a paradigmatic placebo analgesia experiment in the laboratory, participants are placed in a context in which they will receive aversive stimulation (thermal pain, shock, etc.). Participants are given information suggesting that an external agent, such as an injection or an ointment, is a powerful analgesic that will reduce pain. The agent, however, is a pharmacologically inert substance such as saline or starch. Noxious stimulation is presented, and responses to stimulation with placebo are compared with responses to stimulation without placebo. This experimental design allows researchers to examine a variety of variables as indices of pain, including subjective ratings, physiological responses, and pain-related activity in brain regions known to be associated with pain processing. Changes in these pain-related dependent variables in the placebo condition may be attributed to the placebo response.

The same approach can be used to investigate the role of the placebo response in anxiety (placebo anxiolytics paired with aversive images (Petrovic et al. 2005), motor performance in Parkinson's disease (sham stimulation of subthalamic nucleus paired with motor performance (Benedetti et al. 2003; Pollo et al. 2002) or any other relevant biopsychological process that may be elicited and measured in the laboratory.

Through careful manipulations, researchers are able to examine the specific contributions of various factors to the placebo response. Such studies include investigations of the role of the medical context on placebo; researchers have investigated pill characteristics (Blackwell, Bloomfield, and Buncher 1972), effects of branding (Branthwaite and

Cooper 1981), and method of delivery (Levine and Gordon 1984), among other detailed aspects of the medical context (see Barrett et al. 2006 for a review). The role of psychological processes has also been investigated through laboratory experiments. For example, many experimental studies have sought to elucidate the contributions of conscious expectancies and conditioning to the development of placebo responses and to understand whether the two processes act independently or in parallel (Benedetti et al. 2003; I. Kirsch 1985; I. Kirsch 2004; Montgomery and Kirsch 1997; Stewart-Williams and Podd 2004; N. J. Voudouris et al. 1985; N. J. Voudouris, Peck, and Coleman 1989; N. J. Voudouris, Peck, and Coleman 1990).

Many studies have used laboratory experiments to investigate the role of patient characteristics on the placebo effect; for a long time, researchers sought to identify factors that would identify "placebo responders". This effort stemmed from the observation that in nearly every study of the placebo effect, a subgroup of individuals did not respond to placebo manipulations; it was thought that factors could be identified that would determine whether or not an individual would be susceptible to placebo manipulations. Personality traits such as suggestibility were investigated, but no significant relationship was ever convincingly demonstrated. For example, Liberman (1964) wrote, "Placebo reactivity should be viewed as a potential tendency that can become manifest in the right circumstances in anyone rather than as an attribute possessed by some but not by others."

Perhaps most important, laboratory investigations allow researchers to examine the endogenous mechanisms responsible for the placebo effect. Research in both animals and humans has identified neurochemical factors and nervous system pathways subserving endogenous regulation of psychological and physiological endpoints. Researchers have the opportunity to differentiate between mechanisms contributing to placebo effects across domains and domain-specific mechanisms. Understanding these mechanisms can promote scientific understanding of endogenous control processes and mind-body connections as well as shed light on potential targets for clinical intervention.

We have adopted this approach in order to study placebo effects on pain by using neuroimaging methods to examine placebo responses during noxious thermal stimulation. Placebo-elicited reductions in reported pain correlate with decreases in important pain-related brain activity (evidenced through both fMRI and ERPs) and relate inversely to opioid binding (evidenced with PET neurochemical imaging). This provides strong evidence that placebo effects are indeed active psycho-biological processes and not simply reporting biases. We will now review this research to offer evidence of the mechanisms by which placebo responses modulate the pain experience.

Sensory components of pain

Before we discuss our current understanding of the neurobiological mechanisms involved in placebo analgesia and what this can offer us in the way of understanding mind-body connections and endogenous regulation of physiological endpoints, it is important to review the basic physiological architecture underlying pain processing. In the case of pain induced by noxious stimulation, information about this stimulation is first registered by specialized nociceptors below the skin's surface. Even at this level, it is clear that pain is a psychological construct since pain can occur without nociceptor stimulation, and nociceptors stimulation can occur without eliciting pain.

There are two types of primary afferent nociceptors (PANs) that are specialized to transmit information about pain: A and C fibers. These fibers are differentiated by diameter and amount of myelination, which allows them to transmit information about different sorts of pain, with sharp pain information relayed primarily by the larger myelinated A fibers and dull pain transmitted by the slower unmyelinated C-fibers. PANs synapse with neurons in the laminae of the spinal cord's dorsal horn, which then cross to the anterolateral quadrant and form three ascending pathways: the spinothalamic tract, the spinoreticular tract, and the spinomesencephalic tract. Pain signals ascend to cortex via thalamus and brain stem relay centers, including the periaqueductal gray (PAG), rostral ventral medulla (RVM), and nucleus cuneiformis (NCF) (Tracey and Mantyh 2007). Sensory components of pain (intensity and location) are processed initially by primary and secondary somatosensory cortices (SI and SII, respectively). From here, pain signals are distributed further to higher cortical processing areas, such as anterior insula, dorsal and rostral anterior cingulate cortex (ACC), and orbitofrontal cortex (OFC); these regions are thought to play an important role in the affective components of pain (Price 2000).

Thus far, we have reviewed the mechanisms involved in transmitting nociceptive information from peripheral sensation to cortical representation. As a result of research on the ascending pathways, researchers historically viewed pain as a sensory modality, with the main goal of pain to signal potential damage; the brain perceives and responds to nociceptive signals carried by the ascending pathways, the spinal cord is involved only as a relay station, and pain modulation is entirely peripheral.

Pain modulation pathways

Today, we know that the brain constructs pain only partly based on nociceptive input; pain has been found to exist in cases where nociceptive input is impossible, such as phantom pain (Oakley, Whitman, and Halligan 2002) and deafferentation (Hosobuchi 1986), and pain can also occur with light touch or spontaneously. Thus, the brain makes critical decisions about how extensively to process nociceptive input. The brain is not solely responsible for modulatory influences on the transmission of nociceptive information since there are feedback loops at multiple levels of the neuraxis. There are also many cognitive and physiological influences that determine the direction of pain in response to noxious stimulation, which may be mediated by feedback between structures at any level of the pain pathways. Decreased pain sensation may occur due to positive expectancies (Keltner et al. 2006; Koyama, McHaffie, Laurienti, and Coghill 2005), competition for attention (Bantick et al. 2002; Valet et al. 2004), and sympathetic arousal (Drummond, Finch, Skipworth, and Blockey 2001); sensitization may occur as a result of anxiety (Arntz and de Jong 1993; Arntz, Dreessen, and De Jong 1994), central sensitization (Iannetti et al. 2005), or inflammation (Wieseler-Frank, Maier, and Watkins 2005).

In 1965, Melzack and Wall put forth their influential gate control theory (Melzack and Wall 1965), which was the first significant step in research aiming to understand the mechanisms behind descending modulation of pain information. They hypothesized that central control mechanisms interact with afferent information at the level of the spinal cord in order to block nociceptive signals from reaching the thalamus and central nervous system. Subsequent research on the specifics of such modulation has brought us to our current understanding of pain as a CNS phenomenon; in order to understand pain, the brain, responsible for decisions and understanding of context and a powerful source of descending modulation of spinal transmission, cannot be ignored.

We now know that this "gate control" may be achieved through descending endogenous opioids. Endogenous opioids were first implicated in placebo analgesia when the opioid antagonist naloxone, an agent that specifically binds to -opioid receptors, was shown to reverse behavioral placebo effects (Levine, Gordon, and Fields 1978). These results have been replicated (Benedetti, Arduino, and Amanzio 1999; Grevert, Albert, and Goldstein 1983; Levine and Gordon 1984; Levine, Gordon, and Fields 1979), although studies also support nonopioid mechanisms of placebo (Amanzio and Benedetti 1999; Gracely, Dubner, Wolskee, and Deeter 1983; Scott et al. 2007, 2008). The release of these peptides is critically controlled by the periacqueductal gray (PAG) and rostral ventromedial medulla (RVM), and opioids have been shown to have an inhibitory effect on PAN synapses at the level of the spinal cord's dorsal horn (Fields 2004).

Naloxone is also capable of reversing the analgesic effects of direct stimulation of the PAG (Morgan, Gold, Liebeskind, and Stein 1991). Since the PAG is a major center for opioids with the ability to provide both descending modulation of nociception as well as modulation of frontal and limbic circuitry, it is likely to serve a key role in the modulation of pain under placebo. This provides a promising mechanism by which context-dependent regulation of pain may occur, with reciprocal connections between important pain-processing and decision-making areas of cortex and the PAG.

Importantly, PAG has been shown to be under prefrontal control. Frontal cortex activation correlates with reduced across-subjects connectivity between PAG and thalamus (Lorenz, Minoshima, and Casey 2003; Valet et al. 2004). Stimulation of ventrolateral OFC blocks the analgesic effects of PAG stimulation (Zhang, Tang, Yuan, and Jia 1998). Finally, connectivity between rostral ACC and PAG increases under placebo (Bandler and Shipley 1994; Bingel et al. 2006). With the columns of the PAG organized to elicit coordinated behavior (inferior right for flight responses, superior right for fight responses, and left column for withdrawal) (Bandler and Shipley 1994), the PAG may be critical in allowing for frontal contextual information to influence drive state and physiology.

Placebo analgesia

With this background in mind, we can now begin to examine research on pain pathway regulation by placebo-induced cognitive expectancies. We used a placebo manipulation to induce expectations for pain relief during noxious thermal stimulation (Wager et al. 2004). A placebo cream was put on participants' skin with the explanation that it was lidocaine and would have pain-relieving effects. This was compared to a control cream that participants were told would have no effect. Unbeknownst to participants, the two creams were actually identical. Participants reported a 22% decrease in pain with the placebo cream.

With fMRI, we can examine activity in the brain in order to determine where in the pain-processing stream placebos may have their effect. Activation during noxious stimulation is compared between placebo and control trials. Three potential mechanisms exist, which are not necessarily mutually exclusive. First, the placebo response may take place through spinal inhibition, as suggested by the gate control theory; in this case, we would expect to see widespread decreases in responses evoked by noxious stimulation in pain-processing regions, since afferent nociceptive information would be prevented from reaching cortical levels of processing. This possibility is supported by work by Bushnell (Bushnell, Duncan, Dubner, and He 1984), Fields (Fields 2004), and Matre and colleagues (Matre, Casey, and Knardahl 2006).

Alternatively, the placebo response may induce changes in pain affect and central pain processing (Clark 1969; Rainville, Duncan, Price, Carrier et al. 1997), which would lead us to expect decreases in pain response in selected regions only. Finally, placebo treatments may induce changes in reporting bias but leave pain-evoked responses unaffected. This alternative would be manifest during functional imaging as changes in decision-making circuits during or after pain, at which point decisions are made retrospectively as to magnitude of pain during stimulation.

We examined pain processing both during noxious stimulation as well as during the anticipatory period preceding stimulation (Wager et al. 2004). We found that, relative to the control condition, placebo administration did indeed induce decreases in pain-processing regions during painful stimulation. These decreases occurred both in regions associated with sensory-discriminative pain processing (thalamus) as well as in regions known to be responsible for processing the affective components of pain (anterior insula, ACC). These decreases have been replicated (Price, Craggs, Verne, Perlstein et al. 2007), although other research has failed to replicate decreases (Kong et al. 2006).

An important aspect of these results is that most of the observed placebo-induced decreases occurred late in the pain period. These delayed decreases could have resulted either from early inhibition of the pain response, as the gate control theory would suggest, or could have been an artifact of decision-making processes rather than actual pain inhibition. In order to examine fast, early effects of placebo, we conducted a second study in which we used laser-evoked pain (LEP) and ERPs (Wager et al. 2006). We found that placebo expectations decreased a medial frontal P2 component known to be sensitive to laser intensity and pain at 220 ms, too early to be affected by decision-making and report biases (Posner and Boies 1971). Early modulation of pain by expectancy has also been demonstrated in MEG (Lorenz et al. 2005) and electroencephalography (Watson, El-Deredy, Vogt, and Jones 2007). Even early decreases in pain processing such as these still do not conclusively prove that spinal inhibition has occurred, since placebo-induced decreases in *attention* to pain would also result in a reduction in P2 potentials. In fact, we found that P2 LEP placebo differences habituated over the course of the experiment while placebo effects on reported pain did not; this suggests that inhibition alone cannot fully explain observed placebo effects on reported pain.

Furthermore, if the gate control hypothesis were entirely responsible for changes in reported pain based on inhibition of ascending pain, then effects in the brain would be the same as decreasing the pain input by the same difference as changes in reported pain under placebo. Since we can quantify the relationship between P2 and laser intensity, we were able to actually examine this question and found that the extent of decrease in P2 amplitude was less than the difference that would be required in order to elicit the same difference in ratings based on applied pain. In other words, the difference in reported pain between placebo and control was greater than the difference in P2, suggesting that LEP reduction alone was not sufficient to account for reported placebo effects.

Thus, while there is support for early inhibition of nociceptive signals based on the differences in P2 amplitude between placebo and control conditions, the magnitude of these differences is not large enough to entirely explain placebo effects on reported pain. This suggests that there may be important additional mediators of the relationship between placebo-based expectancies and reported pain, such as attention, appraisal, and other cognitive factors.

We also conducted a study using PET molecular imaging in order to examine neurochemical mechanisms of placebo (Wager et al. 2007). Opioids are known to relieve pain, so their involvement in placebo analgesia provides further evidence that placebos recruit powerful endogenous mechanisms to alter pain processing rather than simply affecting decision making and pain reports. Furthermore, in the fMRI experiment reviewed earlier, an area of the midbrain surrounding the PAG was found to be recruited during pain anticipation under placebo and was correlated with right dorsolateral prefrontal cortex (DLPFC). Studying the role of endogenous opioids in placebo analgesia may provide a basis for understanding the mechanisms by which the frontal cortex, known to be involved in higher-level processes such as executive function, expectancy, and evaluation, might modulate pain. We used PET in order to examine opioid binding in placebo during warmth and painful heat. [11C]Carfentinil, a radioactive tracer, binds to opioid receptors, which allows us to infer opioid binding activity: [11C]Carfentinil binding is inversely related to opioid binding, since the two compete for receptor space.

Thus, if we see decreased tracer binding in a region during placebo relative to the control condition, we can infer that endogenous opioid binding has increased under placebo. In general, we assume there is a basic feedback loop between nociception and opioid release, where nociception recruits opioid release in order to inhibit subsequent nociception. Our results suggest that placebo leads to opioid potentiation; placebo modulated reported pain and led to increases in opioid binding during heat but not during nonpainful warmth. Placebo-heat interactions were observed in NRM, PAG, OFC, and rACC, among other pain-responsive regions of interest, and networks of these regions were found to be functionally integrated under placebo. These results help elucidate the critical role of endogenous opioids in the placebo response; opioid release in affective brain regions is potentiated during placebo.

In complementary work, researchers have examined the role of dopamine, a neurotransmitter thought to be highly related to reward, prediction, and learning, in placebo analgesia. Since some have argued that analgesia may be a special case of reward processing—pain relief may be thought to be rewarding in and of itself (Fields 2004; Irizarry and Licinio 2005)—researchers have been interested in examining the contributions of dopamine systems to placebo analgesia. Recent studies have used PET molecular imaging with [^{11}C]raclopride to label dopamine binding during placebo analgesia.

In one study (Scott et al. 2008), researchers directly investigated the connection between opioid and dopamine systems in placebo analgesia by using PET to image both dopamine and opioid receptor binding in the same individuals. Placebo induced increased opioid and dopamine release (reduced tracer binding) in the nucleus accumbens as well as other areas. Dopamine increases in the nucleus accumbens were correlated with opioid increases in the same region as well as with reported placebo analgesia. This provides evidence for the role of dopamine in placebo analgesia and suggests that there may be an important relationship between dopamine and opioid systems in the placebo response. The same group also examined the relationship between placebo analgesia, endogenous opioid release, and reward processing (Scott et al. 2007) and focused on the nucleus accumbens (NAcc), a dopamine-rich part of the basal ganglia's ventral striatum. Dopamine binding in the NAcc during noxious stimulation correlated with anticipated effectiveness of the placebo, and the magnitude of dopamine binding during pain anticipation correlated with the magnitude of placebo effects on reported pain.

In a subsequent fMRI portion of the experiment, participants participated in a monetary reward task; high placebo responders were found to show greater NAcc activity during reward anticipation, and NAcc activity during reward anticipation was correlated with dopamine activity during placebo analgesia. These results provide evidence for a link between placebo analgesia and reward processing.

In conclusion, placebo treatments manipulate cognitive context in order to shape the pain experience. We have presented evidence for an early inhibition component, supported by early LEP effects on pain, and a larger central (limbic) component. Mechanisms of placebo analgesia involve frontal regulation of PAG and limbic system, mediated to a large extent by endogenous opioid release as well as dopamine subsytems.

Extending the findings to other domains

If placebo analgesia is a model system for placebo responses, then what are the principles of placebo responding that may be drawn? In both the fMRI and PET opioid binding studies, the regions that showed the greatest placebo responses were those known to be related to affect and value, such as the insula, rostral ACC, and OFC. For instance, a meta-analysis in our lab (Kober et al. in press) that examined 162 studies of emotion showed that the anterior insula was more consistently activated during various kinds of negative emotional experience than during positive experience. Thus, insula changes need not be specific for pain; they could indicate shifts in emotional experience. Dopamine and NAcc activity, also shown to be involved in placebo analgesia, are also thought to be central for a variety of affective or value-based processes, such as hedonic experiences (pleasure and pain) and the motivated pursuit of goals. In fact, both opioid and dopamine systems have been linked to positive shifts in hedonic processes and appetitive motivation.

Thus, placebo responses may exist (and be strongest) in outcomes that are most directly affected by this evaluation system of the brain. Indeed, placebo effects are also found in other disorders in which emotional evaluation and motivation play a role. One of the most prominent is Major Depressive Disorder (I. Kirsch 1998, 2000; I. Kirsch et al. 2008; Mayberg et al. 2002; Rutherford et al. submitted). For example, Rutherford found that patients assigned to a drug in a clinical trial respond more strongly in comparator trials, in which they are told they will get an active drug for certain, than in double-blind trials, in which they have only a 50% chance of receiving the drug. Mayberg and colleagues (Mayberg et al. 2002) showed that placebo antidepressants affect brain metabolic activity much in the same way as their active pharmacological counterparts, including important changes in subgenual ACC, a region consistently affected in depression and that is the target of deep brain stimulation for treatment-resistant patients.

A second disorder that is perhaps even better understood in terms of its neurobiological bases and the role of the placebo response therein is Parkinson's disease, a movement disorder caused by degeneration of dopamine-producing neurons in the basal ganglia's substantia nigra. Placebo responses in Parkinson's disease have been shown to modulate striatal dopamine release (de la Fuente-Fernandez et al. 2001) and activity in the subthalamic nucleus, a stimulation site used in the treatment of Parkinson's (Benedetti et al. 2004), and expectations for enhanced vs. poor motor performance can modulate the effects of subthalamic nucleus stimulation (Pollo et al. 2002). Dopamine itself is important in motivated behavior (Berridge and Robinson 1998; Schultz, Dayan, and Montague 1997; Smith and Berridge 2005), so it is quite reasonable to view these data in light of placebo responses entailing motivation and appraisal subsystems.

It is even possible to reconcile research that demonstrates placebo responses in physical outcome measures, such as the meta-analysis reviewed earlier (Meissner et al. 2007), with this affective account of placebo responses. Saying something is "physical" does not mean it cannot be susceptible to motivation. In asthma, for example, one measure that has commonly shown placebo effects is FEV-1, or forced expiratory volume (Kemeny et al. 2007; Leigh, MacQueen, Tougas, Hargreave, and Bienenstock 2003). FEV-1 may be influenced by brain stem centers that control respiration, and these brain stem centers are targets of projections from some of the same higher-level regions that showed placebo effects in pain—in particular, the PAG and ventromedial PFC. Thus, to say that placebo effects are related to evaluation and motivation does not imply that they cannot be "real" and have objectively measurable consequences in the body. The central systems most closely associated with appraisal control brain stem circuits that affect all the major organ systems.

In addition, motivation in this sense need not even be conscious. Psychology researchers have demonstrated a wealth of effects of unconsciously processed stimuli on perception and behavior (Bargh, Gollwitzer, Lee-Chai, Barndollar, and Trotschel 2001) (Winkielman, Berridge, and Wilbarger 2005), including potentiating physiological skin conductance responses to fear conditioning (Olsson and Phelps 2004). Fields (Fields 2004) has argued that the core limbic systems of the brain control spinal pain transmission in an adaptive way—decreasing pain under conditions in which it is essential to do so (fight, flight) and increasing it under others, depending on the environmental context.

Our proposal that placebo responses are mediated by changes in affective evaluation is not entirely unrelated to proposals that placebo involves "reward" (de la Fuente-Fernandez et al. 2004; Scott et al.

2007), mentioned in the preceding section. However, saying that reward plays a role in placebo seems a bit akin to saying that changes with placebo are the same as those involved in any manipulation of positive emotion—say, in receiving a bag of candy or finding a five-dollar bill on the ground. In fact, there is not substantial evidence that pain can be affected by these things. The alternative is something more subtle: That placebo changes appraisals of safety and threat depending on the perceived context and beliefs about the placebo treatment, and that these changes in appraisal are mediated by brain circuitry in the limbic system that affects emotion, motivation, and pain. Thus, to ask "Does placebo affect the body or just the brain" may be asking the wrong question. We may instead want to ask, "How does placebo affect the brain, and under what conditions are brain-peripheral pathways affected?"

Summary

Careful experimental manipulations have the power to provide strong evidence of active placebo responses, refuting assertions that placebo effects are nothing but reporting biases and statistical artifacts. Research using placebo analgesia as a model system suggests that placebo responses recruit powerful endogenous processes to modulate perception, and that such modulation may be mediated by changes in affective evaluation. This motivational account is not limited to placebo analgesia, for similar mechanisms have been demonstrated to be involved in placebo responses in Major Depressive Disorder and Parkinson's disease. The cortical and subcortical regions involved in affect and evaluation are indeed able to modulate peripheral outcomes, providing candidate mechanisms that may support placebo responses across a range of disorders and clinical conditions. These placebo response mechanisms are presumably at work in active behavioral and pharmacological therapies as well. These mechanisms elucidated by experimental research on the placebo response thereby provide a powerful window into understanding how the brain is capable of modulating the body's physiological state.

REFERENCES

Amanzio, M., and F. Benedetti. 1999. Neuropharmacological dissection of placebo analgesia: Expectation-activated opioid systems versus conditioning-activated specific subsystems. *J Neurosci* 19(1): 484–494.

Arntz, A., and P. de Jong. 1993. Anxiety, attention and pain. *J Psychosom Res* 37(4): 423–431.

Arntz, A., L. Dreessen, and P. De Jong. 1994. The influence of anxiety on pain: attentional and attributional mediators. *Pain* 56(3): 307–314.

Bandler, R., and M. T. Shipley. 1994. Columnar organization in the midbrain periaqueductal gray: modules for emotional expression? *Trends Neurosci* 17(9): 379–389.

Bantick, S. J., R. G. Wise, A. Ploghaus, S. Clare, S. M. Smith, and I. Tracey. 2002. Imaging how attention modulates pain in humans using functional MRI. *Brain* 125(Pt 2): 310–319.

Bargh, J. A., P.M. Gollwitzer, A. Lee-Chai, K. Barndollar, and R. Trotschel. 2001. The automated will: Nonconscious activation and pursuit of behavioral goals. *J Pers Soc Psychol* 81(6): 1014–1027.

Barrett, B., D. Muller, D. Rakel, D. Rabago, L. Marchand, and J. C. Scheder. 2006. Placebo, meaning, and health. *Perspect Biol Med* 49(2): 178–198.

Benedetti, F. 2007. Placebo and endogenous mechanisms of analgesia. *Handb Exp Pharmacol* (177): 393–413.

Benedetti, F., and M. Amanzio. 1997. The neurobiology of placebo analgesia: From endogenous opioids to cholecystokinin. *Prog Neurobiol* 52(2): 109–125.

Benedetti, F., M. Amanzio, S. Baldi, C. Casadio, A. Cavallo, M. Mancuso, et al. 1998. The specific effects of prior opioid exposure on placebo analgesia and placebo respiratory depression. *Pain* 75(2–3): 313–319.

Benedetti, F., M. Amanzio, S. Baldi, C. Casadio, and G. Maggi. 1999. Inducing placebo respiratory depressant responses in humans via opioid receptors. *Eur J Neurosci* 11(2): 625–631.

Benedetti, F., M. Amanzio, and G. Maggi. 1995. Potentiation of placebo analgesia by proglumide. *Lancet* 346(8984): 1231.

Benedetti, F., M. Amanzio, S. Vighetti, and G. Asteggiano. 2006. The biochemical and neuroendocrine bases of the hyperalgesic nocebo effect. *J Neurosci* 26(46):12014–12022.

Benedetti, F., C. Arduino, and M. Amanzio. 1999. Somatotopic activation of opioid systems by target-directed expectations of analgesia. *J Neurosci* 19(9): 3639–3648.

Benedetti, F., L. Colloca, E. Torre, M. Lanotte, A. Melcarne, M. Pesare, M. et al. 2004. Placebo-responsive Parkinson patients show decreased activity in single neurons of subthalamic nucleus. *Nat Neurosci* 7(6): 587–588.

Benedetti, F., M. Lanotte, L. Lopiano, and L. Colloca. 2007. When words are painful: Unraveling the mechanisms of the nocebo effect. *Neuroscience* 147: 260–271.

Benedetti, F., A. Pollo, L. Lopiano, M. Lanotte, S. Vighetti, and I. Rainero. 2003. Conscious expectation and unconscious conditioning in analgesic, motor, and hormonal placebo/nocebo responses. *J Neurosci* 23(10): 4315–4323.

Berridge, K. C., and T. E. Robinson. 1998. What is the role of dopamine in reward: hedonic impact, reward learning, or incentive salience? *Brain Res Brain Res Rev* 28(3): 309–369.

Bingel, U., J. Lorenz, E. Schoell, C. Weiller, and C. Buchel. 2006. Mechanisms of placebo analgesia: rACC recruitment of a subcortical antinociceptive network. *Pain* 120(1–2): 8–15.

Blackwell, B., S. S. Bloomfield, and C. R. Buncher. 1972. Demonstration to medical students of placebo responses and non-drug factors. *Lancet* 1(7763): 1279–1282.

Branthwaite, A., and P. Cooper. 1981. Analgesic effects of branding in treatment of headaches. *British medical journal (Clinical research ed.)* 282(6276): 1576–1578.

Bushnell, M. C., G. H. Duncan, R. Dubner, and L. F. He. 1984. Activity of trigeminothalamic neurons in medullary dorsal horn of awake monkeys trained in a thermal discrimination task. *J. Neurophysiol.* 52: 170–187.

Clark, W. C. 1969. Sensory-decision theory analysis of the placebo effect on the criterion for pain and thermal sensitivity. *J Abnorm Psychol* 74(3): 363–371.

Colloca, L., L. Lopiano, M. Lanotte, and F. Benedetti. 2004. Overt versus covert treatment for pain, anxiety, and Parkinson's disease. *Lancet Neurol* 3(11): 679–684.

de la Fuente-Fernandez, R., T. J. Ruth, V. Sossi, M. Schulzer, D. B. Calne, and A. J. Stoessl. 2001. Expectation and dopamine release: Mechanism of the placebo effect in Parkinson's disease. *Science* 293(5532): 1164–1166.

de la Fuente-Fernandez, R., M. Schulzer, and A. J. Stoessl. 2004. Placebo mechanisms and reward circuitry: clues from Parkinson's disease. *Biol Psychiatry* 56(2): 67–71.

De Pascalis, V., C. Chiaradia, and E. Carotenuto. 2002. The contribution of suggestibility and expectation to placebo analgesia phenomenon in an experimental setting. *Pain* 96(3): 393–402.

Drummond, P. D., P. M. Finch, S. Skipworth, and P. Blockey. 2001. Pain increases during sympathetic arousal in patients with complex regional pain syndrome. *Neurology* 57(7):1296–1303.

Fields, H. 2004. State-dependent opioid control of pain. *Nat Rev Neurosci* 5(7): 565–575.

Goebel, M. U., N. Meykadeh, W. Kou, M. Schedlowski, and U. R. Hengge. (In press.). Behavioral Conditioning of Antihistamine Effects in Patients with Allergic Rhinitis. *Psychotherapy and Psychosomatics.*

Goebel, M. U., A. E. Trebst, J. Steiner, Y. F. Xie, M. S. Exton, S. Frede et al. 2002. Behavioral conditioning of immunosuppression is possible in humans. *Faseb J* 16(14): 1869–1873.

Gracely, R. H., R. Dubner, P. J. Wolskee, and W. R. Deeter. 1983. Placebo and naloxone can alter post-surgical pain by separate mechanisms. *Nature* 306(5940): 264–265.

Grevert, P., L. H. Albert, and A. Goldstein. 1983. Partial antagonism of placebo analgesia by naloxone. *Pain* 16(2): 129–143.

Hall, M. A., E. Dugan, B. Zheng, and A. K. Mishra. 2001. Trust in physicians and medical institutions: What is it, can it be measured, and does it matter? *The Milbank Quarterly* 79(4): 613–639.

Harrington, A., ed. 1999. *The placebo effect.* Cambridge, MA: Harvard University Press.

Hosobuchi, Y. 1986. Subcortical electrical stimulation for control of intractable pain in humans. Report of 122 cases (1970–1984). *J Neurosurg* 64(4): 543–553.

Hrobjartsson, A., and P. C. Gotzsche. 2001. Is the placebo powerless? An analysis of clinical trials comparing placebo with no treatment. *New England Journal of Medicine,* 344(21): 1594–1602.

Hrobjartsson, A., and P. C. Gotzsche. 2004. Is the placebo powerless? Update of a systematic review with 52 new randomized trials comparing placebo with no treatment. *J Intern Med* 256(2): 91–100.

Iannetti, G. D., L. Zambreanu, R. G. Wise, T. J. Buchanan, J. P. Huggins, T. S. Smart et al. 2005. Pharmacological modulation of pain-related brain activity during normal and central sensitization states in humans. *Proc Natl Acad Sci U S A* 102(50): 18195–18200.

Irizarry, K. J., and J. Licinio. 2005. An explanation for the placebo effect? *Science* 307(5714): 1411–1412.

Johansen, O., J. Brox, and M. A. Flaten. 2003. Placebo and Nocebo responses, cortisol, and circulating beta-endorphin. *Psychosom Med* 65(5):786–790.

Keltner, J. R., A. Furst, C. Fan, R. Redfern, B. Inglis, and H. L. Fields. 2006. Isolating the modulatory effect of expectation on pain transmission: a functional magnetic resonance imaging study. *J Neurosci* 26(16): 4437–4443.

Kemeny, M. E., L. J. Rosenwasser, R. A. Panettieri, R. M. Rose, S. M. Berg-Smith, and J. N. Kline. 2007. Placebo response in asthma: a robust and objective phenomenon. *J Allergy Clin Immunol* 119(6): 1375–1381.

Kienle, G. S., and H. Kiene. 1997. The powerful placebo effect: fact or fiction? *J Clin Epidemiol* 50(12): 1311–1318.

Kirsch, I. 1985. Response expectancy as a determinant of experience and behavior. *American Psychologist* 40: 1189–1202.

Kirsch, I. 1998. Listening to Prozac but hearing placebo: A meta-analysis of antidepressant medication. *Prevention & Treatment* 1.

Kirsch, I. 2000. Are drug and placebo effects in depression additive? *Biol Psychiatry* 47(8): 733–735.

Kirsch, I. 2004. Conditioning, expectancy, and the placebo effect: Comment on Stewart-Williams and Podd. *Psychol Bull* 130(2): 341–343.

Kirsch, I., B. J. Deacon, T. B. Huedo-Medina, A. Scoboria, T. J. Moore, and B. T. Johnson. 2008. Initial severity and antidepressant benefits: A meta-analysis of data submitted to the Food and Drug Administration. *PLoS Med* 5(2): e45.

Kirsch, I., and A. Scoboria. 2001. Apples, oranges, and placebos: Heterogeneity in a meta-analysis of placebo effects. *Adv Mind Body Med* 17(4): 307–309; discussion 312–308.

Kober, H., L. Barrett, J. Joseph, E. Bliss-Moreau, K. Lindquist, and T. Wager. (In press). Functional grouping and cortical-subcortical interactions in emotion: A meta-analysis of neuroimaging studies. *NeuroImage*.

Kong, J., R. L. Gollub, I. S. Rosman, J. M. Webb, M. G. Vangel, I. Kirsch et al. 2006. Brain activity associated with expectancy-enhanced placebo analgesia as measured by functional magnetic resonance imaging. *J Neurosci* 26(2): 381–388.

Koyama, T., J. G. McHaffie, P. J. Laurienti, and R. C. Coghill. 2005. The subjective experience of pain: Where expectations become reality. *Proc Natl Acad Sci U S A* 102(36): 12950–12955.

Kradin, R. L. 2004. The placebo response: its putative role as a functional salutogenic mechanism of the central nervous system. *Perspect Biol Med* 47(3): 328–338.

Lanotte, M., L. Lopiano, E. Torre, B. Bergamasco, L. Colloca, and F. Benedetti. 2005. Expectation enhances autonomic responses to stimulation of the human subthalamic limbic region. *Brain Behav Immun* 19(6): 500–509.

Leigh, R., G. MacQueen, G. Tougas, F. E. Hargreave, and J. Bienenstock. 2003. Change in forced expiratory volume in 1 second after sham bronchoconstrictor in suggestible but not suggestion-resistant asthmatic subjects: A pilot study. *Psychosom Med* 65(5): 791–795.

Levine, J. D., and N. C. Gordon. 1984. Influence of the method of drug administration on analgesic response. *Nature* 312(5996): 755–756.

Levine, J. D., N. C. Gordon, and H. L. Fields. 1978. The mechanism of placebo analgesia. *Lancet* 2(8091): 654–657.

Levine, J. D., N. C. Gordon, and H. L. Fields. 1979. Naloxone dose dependently produces analgesia and hyperalgesia in postoperative pain. *Nature* 278(5706): 740–741.

Liberman, R. 1964. An experimental study of the placebo response under three different situations of pain. *J Psychiatr Res.* 2: 233–246.

Lorenz, J., M. Hauck, R. C. Paur, Y. Nakamura, R. Zimmermann, B. Bromm et al. 2005. Cortical correlates of false expectations during pain intensity judgments--a possible manifestation of placebo/nocebo cognitions. *Brain Behav Immun* 19(4): 283–295.

Lorenz, J., S. Minoshima, and K. L. Casey. 2003. Keeping pain out of mind: The role of the dorsolateral prefrontal cortex in pain modulation. *Brain* 126(Pt 5): 1079–1091.

Matre, D., K. L. Casey, and S. Knardahl. 2006. Placebo-induced changes in spinal cord pain processing. *J Neurosci* 26(2): 559–563.

Mayberg, H. S., J. A. Silva, S. K. Brannan, J. L.Tekell, R. K. Mahurin, S. McGinnis et al. 2002. The functional neuroanatomy of the placebo effect. *Am J Psychiatry* 159(5): 728–737.

Meissner, K., H. Distel, and U. Mitzdorf. 2007. Evidence for placebo effects on physical but not on biochemical outcome parameters: a review of clinical trials. *BMC Med* 5: 3.

Melzack, R., and P. D. Wall. 1965. Pain mechanisms: A new theory. *Science* 150(699): 971–979.

Moerman, D. E., and W. B. Jonas. 2002. Deconstructing the placebo effect and finding the meaning response. *Ann Intern Med* 136(6): 471–476.

Montgomery, G. H., and I. Kirsch. 1997. Classical conditioning and the placebo effect. *Pain* 72(1-2): 107–113.

Morgan, M. M., M. S. Gold, J. C. Liebeskind, and C. Stein. 1991. Periaqueductal gray stimulation produces a spinally mediated, opioid antinociception for the inflamed hindpaw of the rat. *Brain Res* 545(1–2): 17–23.

Moseley, J. B., Jr., N. P. Wray, D. Kuykendall, K. Willis, and G. Landon. 1996. Arthroscopic treatment of osteoarthritis of the knee: A prospective, randomized, placebo-controlled trial. Results of a pilot study. *Am J Sports Med* 24(1): 28–34.

Oakley, D. A., L. G. Whitman, and P. W. Halligan. 2002. Hypnotic imagery as a treatment for phantom limb pain: Two case reports and a review. *Clin Rehabil* 16(4): 368–377.

Olsson, A., and E. A. Phelps. 2004. Learned fear of "unseen" faces after Pavlovian, observational, and instructed fear. *Psychological Science /APS* 15(12): 822–828.

Petrovic, P., T. Dietrich, P. Fransson, J. Andersson, K. Carlsson, and M. Ingvar. 2005. Placebo in emotional processing-induced expectations of anxiety relief activate a generalized modulatory network. *Neuron* 46(6): 957–969.

Petrovic, P., E. Kalso, K. M. Petersson, and M. Ingvar. 2002. Placebo and opioid analgesia—imaging a shared neuronal network. *Science* 295(5560): 1737–1740.

Pollo, A., E. Torre, L. Lopiano, M. Rizzone, M. Lanotte, A. Cavanna et al. 2002. Expectation modulates the response to subthalamic nucleus stimulation in Parkinsonian patients. *Neuroreport* 13(11): 1383–1386.

Pollo, A., S. Vighetti, I. Rainero, and F. Benedetti. (2003). Placebo analgesia and the heart. *Pain* 102(1–2): 125–133.

Posner, M. I., and S. J. Boies. 1971. Components of attention. *Psychological Review* 78(5): 391–408.

Price, D. D. 2000. Psychological and neural mechanisms of the affective dimension of pain. *Science* 288(5472): 1769–1772.

Price, D. D., J. Craggs, G. N. Verne, W. M. Perlstein, and M. E. Robinson. 2007. Placebo analgesia is accompanied by large reductions in pain-related brain activity in irritable bowel syndrome patients. *Pain* 127(1–2): 63–72.

Price, D. D., L. S. Milling, I. Kirsch, A. Duff, G. H. Montgomery, and S. S. Nicholls. 1999. An analysis of factors that contribute to the magnitude of placebo analgesia in an experimental paradigm. *Pain* 83(2): 147–156.

Rainville, P., G. H. Duncan, D. D. Price, B. Carrier et al.. 1997. Pain affect encoded in human anterior cingulate but not somatosensory cortex. *Science* 277: 968–971.

Rutherford, B. R., J. R. Sneed, and S. P. Roose. Does study design influence outcome? The effects of placebo control and treatment duration in antidepressant trials. *Psychotherapy and Psychosomatics* (in press).

Schultz, W., P. Dayan, and P. R. Montague. 1997. A neural substrate of prediction and reward. *Science* 275(5306): 1593–1599.

Scott, D. J., C. S. Stohler, C. M. Egnatuk, H. Wang, R. A. Koeppe, and J. K. Zubieta.

2007. Individual differences in reward responding explain placebo-induced expectations and effects. *Neuron* 55(2): 325–336.

Scott, D. J., C. S. Stohler, C. M. Egnatuk, H. Wang, R. A. Koeppe, and J. K. Zubieta. 2008. Placebo and nocebo effects are defined by opposite opioid and dopaminergic responses. *Arch Gen Psychiatry* 65(2): 220–231.

Shapiro, A. K., and L. A. Morris. 1978. The placebo effect in medical and psychological therapies. In S. L. Garfield and A. E. Bergins, eds., *Handbook of Psychotherapy and Behavior Change: An Empirical Analysis*, 37–55). New York: Aldine Publishing.

Shapiro, A. K., and E. Shapiro. 1999. The placebo: Is it much ado about nothing? In A. Harrington, ed., *The placebo effect*, 12–36. Cambridge, MA: Harvard University Press.

Sherman, R., and J. Hickner. 2008. Academic physicians use placebos in clinical practice and believe in the mind-body connection. *J Gen Intern Med* 23(1): 7–10.

Smith, K. S., and K. C. Berridge. 2005. The ventral pallidum and hedonic reward: Neurochemical maps of sucrose "liking" and food intake. *J Neurosci* 25(38): 8637–8649.

Stewart-Williams, S., and J. Podd. 2004. The placebo effect: dissolving the expectancy versus conditioning debate. *Psychol Bull* 130(2): 324–340.

Storms, M. D., and R. E. Nisbett. 1970. Insomnia and the attribution process. *J Pers Soc Psychol* 16(2): 319–328.

Tracey, I., and P. W. Mantyh. 2007. The cerebral signature for pain perception and its modulation. *Neuron* 55(3): 377–391.

Valet, M., T. Sprenger, H. Boecker, F. Willoch, E. Rummeny, B. Conrad, B. et al. 2004. Distraction modulates connectivity of the cingulo-frontal cortex and the midbrain during pain—an fMRI analysis. *Pain* 109(3): 399–408.

Vase, L., J. L. Riley 3rd, and D. D. Price. 2002. A comparison of placebo effects in clinical analgesic trials versus studies of placebo analgesia. *Pain* 99: 453–452.

Vase, L., M. E. Robinson, G. N. Verne, and D. D. Price. 2005. Increased placebo analgesia over time in irritable bowel syndrome (IBS) patients is associated with desire and expectation but not endogenous opioid mechanisms. *Pain* 115(3): 338–347.

Voudouris, N. J., Peck, C. L., & Coleman, G. (1985). Conditioned placebo responses. *J Pers Soc Psychol*, 48(1), 47-53.

Voudouris, N. J., C. L. Peck, and G. Coleman. 1989. Conditioned response models of placebo phenomena: further support. *Pain* 38: 109–116.

Voudouris, N. J., C. L. Peck, and G. Coleman. 1990. The role of conditioning and verbal expectancy in the placebo response. *Pain* 43(1): 121–128.

Wager, T. D., D. Matre, and K. L. Casey. 2006. Placebo effects in laser-evoked pain potentials. *Brain Behav Immun* 20(3): 219–230.

Wager, T. D., J. K. Rilling, E. E. Smith, A. Sokolik, K. L. Casey, R. J. Davidson et al. 2004. Placebo-induced changes in FMRI in the anticipation and experience of pain. *Science* 303(5661): 1162–1167.

Wager, T. D., D. J. Scott, D. J., and J. K. Zubieta. 2007. Placebo effects on human -opioid activity during pain. *Proc Natl Acad Sci U S A* 104(26): 11056–11061.

Watson, A., W. El-Deredy, B. A. Vogt, and A. K. Jones. 2007. Placebo analgesia is not due to compliance or habituation: EEG and behavioural evidence. *NeuroReport* 18(8): 771–775.

Wieseler-Frank, J., S. F. Maier, and L. R. Watkins. 2005. Immune-to-brain communication dynamically modulates pain: physiological and pathological consequences. *Brain Behav Immun* 19(2): 104–111.

Wilkins, W. 1985. Placebo controls and concepts in chemotherapy and psychotherapy research. In L. White, B. Tursky, and G. E. Shwartz, eds., *Placebo: Theory, research, and mechanisms*. New York: Guilford Press.

Winkielman, P., K. C. Berridge, and J. L. Wilbarger. 2005. Unconscious affective reactions to masked happy versus angry faces influence consumption behavior and judgments of value. *Pers Soc Psychol Bull* 31(1): 121–135.

Zhang, S., J.S. Tang, B. Yuan, and H. Jia. 1998. Inhibitory effects of electrical stimulation of ventrolateral orbital cortex on the rat jaw-opening reflex. *Brain Res* 813(2):359–366.

Zubieta, J. K., J. A. Bueller, L. R. Jackson, D. J. Scott, Y. Xu, R. A. Koeppe et al. 2005. Placebo effects mediated by endogenous opioid activity on mu-opioid receptors. *J Neurosci* 25(34): 7754–7762.

Zubieta, J. K., W. Y. Yau, D. J. Scott, and C. S. Stohler. 2006. Belief or need? Accounting for individual variations in the neurochemistry of the placebo effect. *Brain Behav Immun* 20(1): 15–26.

7

How the Mind and the Brain Co-Create Each Other Daily

Mind-Brain-Gene Research on the Foundations of Consciousness, Creativity, Imagination, and Psychotherapy

ERNEST LAWRENCE ROSSI
AND KATHRYN LANE ROSSI

1. Mirror Neurons and the Mind-Gene Connection in Psychotherapy

The eternal mystery of how consciousness and nature seemingly reflect each other in the mirror of the human mind was the essence of the Woodman/Rossi dialogues in the Blossoms Bloom in the Fire Conference at Pacifica Graduate Institute in Carpinteria in 2006 (Rossi 2007). We discussed a new neuroscience approach to Carl Jung's (1918/1966) synthetic approach to mind-body healing and psychotherapy. We presumed to boldly go where no one had gone before in outlining the newly emerging field of "the bioinformatics of art, beauty, truth, and creativity in psychotherapy." Figure 1 is a very broadly sketched overview of how the mind updates the brain daily via the mirror neuron system encoding the novel and numinous experiences of consciousness and dreaming (Rossi 2007).

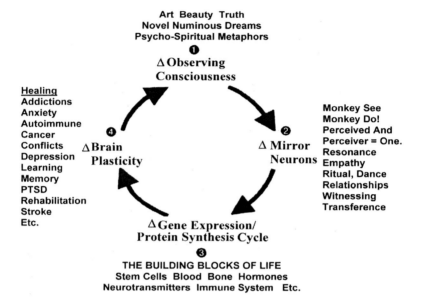

Figure 1: *A neuroscience model of how the mind and brain daily co-create each other. Novel and numinous experiences of (1) observing consciousness can (2) activate mirror neurons to (3) turn on their gene expression/protein synthesis cycle and (4) brain plasticity, which generate the possibility of new consciousness, mind-body healing, and rehabilitation. The delta sign (triangle) means that a change at any of these four levels generates a mathematical transformation to the next level in iterating the recursive cycles of human experience and healing from mind to gene. The outer labels suggest some of the* Psychospiritual Metaphors and Experiences *during Marion Woodman's workshops that may mobilize* the Building Blocks of Life *to facilitate* Mind-Body Healing.

Initial research on the discovery of mirror neurons by Rizzolatti and Arbib (1998) and his research team at the University of Parma in Italy during the early 1990s was described by Miller (2005) as follows:

> The finding was exciting, Rizzolatti says, because it fit with ideas that were coming together at the time in philosophy and cognitive science, such as the hypothesis that understanding the behavior of others involves translating actions we observe into the neural language of our own actions. The monkey mirror neurons seemed to do just that, providing a potential neural mechanism to support that proposal. Subsequently, researchers used functional magnetic resonance imaging (fMRI) and other techniques to investigate brain activity as people made—and observed others making—*hand movements and facial expressions.*

These studies identified mirror-like activity in several regions of the human brain, including a region of frontal cortex homologous to F5. This human frontal region, known as *Broca's area, is also involved in speech production—a connection that snared the attention of researchers studying the evolution of language. . . .* Rizzolatti and others have argued that mirror neurons could facilitate the imitation of skilled movements like t*he hand and mouth movements used for communication . . .* the mirror system in the frontal cortex is active as novices learn to play chords on a guitar by watching a professional guitarist. Similar learning by imitation is a key feature of language acquisition in infants and is widely considered *a prerequisite for language evolution.* (946, emphasis added)

In retrospect we can now see that the excitement about the frontal cortex mirror neuron concept was because it was the first to demonstrate convincingly how specialized neurons not only interface with the outer psychosocial environment but how that interface generates mirroring psychophysiological activity within the brain and body of the observer (Fogassi et al. 2005; Gallese et al. 1996; Iacoboni et al. 2005). Figure 1 outlines my *theoretical neuroscience model* of how novel and numinous experiences of our observing consciousness update and reconstruct the brain at the levels of gene expression and brain plasticity within mirror neurons. This model is speculative and controversial, however, because no one has yet directly demonstrated how activity-dependent gene expression and brain plasticity are actually generated in the F5 region of the human cortex, which is the brain region originally identified as containing mirror neurons defined by Rizzolatti's research team. My theoretical model is, however, entirely consistent with the Nobel Prize-winning research of Eric Kandel (2006), who first described the relationship between activity-dependent gene expression, brain plasticity, and psychotherapy as follows (Kandel 1998):

Insofar as psychotherapy or counseling is effective and produces long-term changes in behavior, it presumably does so through learning, by producing changes in gene expression that alter the strength of synaptic connections and structural changes that alter the anatomical pattern of interconnections between nerve cells of the brain. As the resolution of brain imaging increases, it should eventually permit quantitative evaluation of the outcome of psychotherapy . . . Stated simply, the regulation of gene expression by social factors makes all bodily functions, including all functions of the brain, susceptible to social influences. These social influences will be biologically incorporated in the altered expressions of specific genes in specific nerve cells of specific regions of the brain. These socially influenced alterations are transmitted culturally. They are not incorporated in the sperm and egg and therefore are not transmitted genetically. (460, emphasis added)

The value of adding Kandel's concept of activity-dependent gene expression and brain plasticity to Rizzolatti's mirror neuron concept is that it avoids the problem of infinite regress implied in the mirror concept of mind and consciousness. Rizzolatti uses the concept of the mirror as a metaphor of how the mind works. *But in reality there are no physical mirrors in the mind or brain!* Many brain neurons, however, do respond to novel, salient, and numinous psychological experiences by turning on activity-dependent gene expression and brain plasticity to construct and reconstruct new neural networks that encode images, memories, words, concepts, etc., which actually are the contents of consciousness that function as metaphorical mirrors or windows to the outside world (Rossi 2007).

A generation before Rizzolatti's research on how consciousness seems to mirror and internalize the *outside world*, I conceptualized how our dreams function as a *"self-reflective apparatus"* that mirrors our *internal world* (Rossi 1972/1985/2000). At that time I described this internal mirror neuron system as a "self-reflective apparatus" that could account for two basic categories of dreams I was learning to distinguish in my college student clients: (1) the more common "experiential dreams" in which the dreamer experienced the dream as a vivid here-and-now drama that was really happening, versus (2) the "observer dreams" wherein the dreamer observed herself in a dream drama. Alan Moffit's research team at the Sleep Laboratory in the Department of Psychology at Carleton University in Canada then developed a nine-point *Dream Self-Reflectiveness Scale* to quantify my phenomenological observations on experiential and observer dreams (Moffit 1994; Moffit et al. 1988, 1982). This scale was constructed as a developmental tool to study the evolution of consciousness in dreams (see table 1).

TABLE 1: DREAM SELF-REFLECTIVENESS CATEGORIES
(ROSSI 1972/1985/2000)

1. Dreamer not in dream; objects unfamiliar; no people present.

2. Dreamer not in dream; people or familiar objects present.

3. Dreamer completely involved in dream drama; no self-perspective.

4. Dreamer present predominantly as an observer.

5. Dreamer talks over an idea or has communication with someone.

6. Dreamer undergoes a transformation of body, role, age, emotion, etc.

7. Dreamer has multiple levels of awareness; simultaneously participates in dream drama and observes it. Notices oddities while dreaming; experiences a dream within a dream.

8. Dreamer has significant control in, or control over, dream story; can wake up deliberately.

9. Dreamer can consciously reflect on the fact that he/she is dreaming; lucid dreaming.

A corresponding *Daytime Self-Reflectiveness Scale* (see table 2) was constructed as well by Moffit's student, Susan Purcell (1987; Purcell et al. 1984, 1985, 1986, 1993).

TABLE 2: DAYTIME SELF-REFLECTIVENESS CATEGORIES
(ROSSI 1972/1985/2000)

1. While performing the task, attention is focused on a scene with no people in it (e.g., "watching the screen and the bullets wiping out the ships").

2. While performing the task, attention is focused primarily on a scene with people and/or things that are familiar but without awareness of self (e.g., "these two people are in love, and they want to be together, but people are interfering in their relationship").

3. The person is completely involved with tasks or ambitions that command all attention (e.g., "I was watching the show; I was really involved in it").

4. The person is involved in the task and also watches passively (e.g., "I was watching this soap opera, and this girl is in a hospital bed, and her coach and another lady come in to visit her").

5. While performing the task, the person thinks over an idea and/or thinks over an interaction that involves someone else, involving words and/or definite communication (e.g., "I was thinking about my sister yelling at me in the morning for borrowing her sweater").

6. The person tries to take on the role of another person or undergoes a personal transformation, for example as a different age, a different character(s), as a change of state (from sick to healthy, from human to animal) (e.g., "I thought how pleased I was when I got the score; then I thought I must be nervous because my mouth was dry").

7. The person has multiple perspectives on self, participating and watching at the same time. Noticing something unusual, odd, or bizarre, imagining the loss of consciousness or dying while still watching the scene (e.g., "I was sitting here thinking about falling asleep and what a great room this would be to have as a bedroom").

8. Something in the experience is not right, so the person tries to change it: deliberately stopping thinking about something; removing oneself from an unpleasant experience; deliberately falling asleep in response to an unpleasant experience (e.g., "I started to think about the time my boyfriend got all dressed up and took me to a really nice restaurant for our first anniversary; it was really romantic and then thoughts of the fight we had yesterday kept coming into my mind, so I decided not to let them stay and moved my thoughts back to the fond memory").

9. While involved in the task, the person realizes it is only a dream or an experiment, is transitory, not real in any absolute sense, and may proceed to direct the experience/task (e.g., "I was getting really frustrated with the video game, and suddenly I realized that this was only an experiment and that it doesn't really matter how well I do").

The exciting proposal of this chapter is that these psychological scales of our internal mirror neuron system of self-reflection can now be used by a new generation of students and researchers for assessment of the development of consciousness and creativity in dreams, everyday life, and psychotherapy at the deep psychobiological levels of gene expression and brain plasticity. How to actually do such research into the foundations of mind-gene psychotherapy requires a new vision of how it can be conducted with the million dollar *in silico* databases that are available free on the Internet.

2. A NEW *IN SILICO* MODEL OF RESEARCH IN CONSCIOUSNESS, CREATIVITY, IMAGINATION, PSYCHOTHERAPY, AND MEDICINE: THE NEW COMPUTER ALCHEMY WITHOUT CHEMICALS AND TEST TUBES

In the best of all possible worlds it seems obvious that each of the therapeutic arts and sciences would have an equal share of funding and governmental and academic support. In our real world, however, it is ever more obvious that this is not the case now and probably will never be. Our medical-biological-pharmaceutical industrial complex is able to command billions of dollars annually for new technology and research. Neuroscience, by contrast, manages to get by on hundreds of millions a year. Psychotherapy is scarcely a blip on this radar with only a few million in a good year. In this chapter I propose a new method of *in silico* conceptual research in psychotherapy and medicine that takes an initial step toward equalizing this uneven distribution of research funding and resources by utilizing the million dollar databases of biology that are available free to all on the Internet.

In silico is a popular expression in the biological, computer, and bioinformatic sciences to describe simulations of life processes on all levels, from mind and behavior to genomics. These simulations of complex life processes are performed via information processing models *on silicon chips* in computers as a more economical approach to experimentation. *In silico* research is the key to data mining: the exploration, assessment, and integration of the meaning and implications of the research literature in many biological and psychological disciplines that cannot be integrated in any other way. Such *interdisciplinary in silico research* is possible because our current genomic revolution has made the concept of information the common denominator of all the databases in the life sciences.

The Allen Brain Atlas (ABA) is one such database recently assembled at the cost of $100 million, which is now being made available free to anyone with access to the Internet via a personal computer. The ABA will make it possible to integrate medicine, neuroscience, and bioinformatics to shed light on how activity-dependent gene expression is associated with brain development, dysfunctions and therapies of mental illness, psychosocial stress, memory, learning, behavior, cognition, and consciousness itself (Rossi 2007).

Let us now explore how the ABA of gene expression can be utilized to facilitate the theory, research, and practice of psychotherapy and medicine in the near future by students and faculty of graduate schools of psychology (such as Pacifica Graduate Institute) who do not yet have multimillion dollar laboratories of molecular-genomics and neuroscience on campus. *In silico research is the great equalizer in all interdisciplinary research exploring mind-gene communication in psychotherapy and complementary medicine.*

The New Allen Brain Atlas of Gene Expression

The ABA (http://www.brain-map.org) is available free as a web-based database showing the location and activity level of approximately 23,000 genes in the mouse brain, which shares about 90% homology (similarity) with the human brain. Plans are now underway for making a complete human brain atlas of gene expression. This anatomical reference for understanding the role of gene expression for approximately 50 million Americans suffering from brain dysfunctions such as Alzheimer's, epilepsy, and Parkinson's as well as addiction, depression, and stress is already being described as the foundation for a new neuroscience of mind and behavior. In the ABA the data of 250,000 microscope slides, a million brain sections, and 85 million anatomical photo files are assembled for viewing gene expression in three-dimensional cross sections of the brain.

An initial surprising finding revealed by the ABA is that approximately 80% of genes are expressed in brain cells. The high-resolution digital microscopy images of the ABA show the exact location of the genes in brain tissues and cells that are expressed (turned on) to produce the proteins for carrying out all biological functions of mind and behavior in health and dysfunction.

At the present time research and publications involving the ABA (http://www.brainatlas.org/aba/) are still dominated by biology and medical applications. Of particular interest for psychotherapy, however, is the ABA potential for exploring genes expressed during brain plasticity (synaptogenesis and neurogenesis) in response to normal memory, learning, and behavior, stress-induced dysfunctions, as well as any form of cognitive-behavioral therapy whose effects can be located in the brain by fMRI (Liu et al. 2007; Wang et al. 2006).

Researchers in psychology have been slow in recognizing the implications of activity-dependent gene expression and brain plasticity for the practical applications of psychotherapy because, until now, there has been no obvious and simple way of assessing these deep biological genomic sources of cognition, emotion, and behavior. Gene expression is usually measured by complex and very expensive laboratory procedures, such as DNA microarrays that involve taking invasive tissue samples from the brain, blood, saliva, and body (Rossi 2004, 2007; Rossi et al. 2006). Such invasive procedures have never appeared to be appropriate for assessing psychotherapy in any form. This stumbling block motivates us to outline how the ABA in association with other currently available technologies can enable us to bypass these invasive biological methods with new *in silico* models of exploring the mind-gene connection in all forms of psychotherapy.

Figure 2 outlines how the bioinformatic technologies of the ABA, functional magnetic resonance imaging (fMRI) (Siegel et al. 2006), and the Connectivity Map (Lamb et al. 2006) can be integrated into a new *in silico* model of the theory, research, and practice of psychotherapy by students, researchers, and psychotherapists with nothing more than a personal computer and an Internet connection. This type of *in silico* data mining of existing scientific literature, which I am now proposing for a new conceptual approach to research in psychotherapy, was originally described in a more limited biological context by Blagosklonny and Pardee (2002) as follows:

> Millions of easily retrievable facts are being accumulated in databases, from a variety of sources in seemingly unrelated fields, and from thousands of journals. New knowledge can be generated by "reviewing" these accumulated results in a concept-driven manner, linking them into testable chains and networks . . . Connecting separate facts into new concepts is analogous to combining the 26 letters of the alphabet into languages. One can generate enormous diversity without inventing new letters. These concepts (words), in turn, constitute pieces of more complex concepts (sentences, paragraphs, chapters, books). *We call this process "conceptual" research, to distinguish it from automated data-mining and from conventional theoretical biology.* . . . Can a review provide new knowledge? A review can constitute a comprehensive summary of the data in the field—this type of writing educates but does not directly generate new knowledge. *But a "conceptual" review, on the other hand, can generate knowledge by revealing "cryptic" data and testing hypotheses by published experiments* . . . Conceptual biology *[and psychotherapy]* should

be recognized and criteria established for its publications — new, testable conclusions, supported by published data. In *[psycho]*biological systems, everything is interconnected, and ostensibly unrelated fields are related —the separation of biology into different disciplines is artificial. Conceptual research *[in psychotherapy]* can encompass many fields without limitation. *In comparison with labour-based research, conceptual research is more cost-effective; indeed, verification of a hypothesis using existing data does not limit research to scientists in well-resourced fields or countries.* Hypothesis-driven, experimental research will continue to be a cornerstone of biology, but it should strike up a partnership with the essential components of theoretical and conceptual research [in psychotherapy]." (373, emphasis added)

As can be seen in figure 2, *in silico* conceptual research proceeds in four steps when applied to psychotherapy to discover new associations that may never have been considered by the original laboratory researchers, who first published their data in an apparently unrelated field of pure biology, bioinformatics, genomics, neuroscience, etc.

I illustrate an *in silico* approach to explore how scientific data on the molecular-genomics of psychotherapy can proceed with nothing more than a home computer and an Internet connection in figure 2. Figure 2 illustrates the circular biofeedback flow of information between mind and gene, which is the neuroscientific basis of the transformations of consciousness, creativity, imagination, and healing in psychotherapy and medicine. A full appreciation of the implications of this *in silico* approach for current and future development of the theory, research, and practice of mind-gene psychotherapy proceeds from a comparison of figures 1 and 2.

Figure 1 is a *theoretical neuroscience model* of how the novel and numinous experiences of observing consciousness updates and reconstructs the brain on a daily and hourly basis via mirror neurons.

Figure 2 is a practical *in silico model* of how everyone who knows how to access the Internet with an ordinary home computer can actually do mind-gene research in psychotherapy with existing free databases.

Theoretically one could win a Nobel Prize for doing original research with a home computer utilizing the best peer-reviewed mind-gene research published in our most highly cited peer-reviewed scientific journals. But can all this really be true? Can we really explore

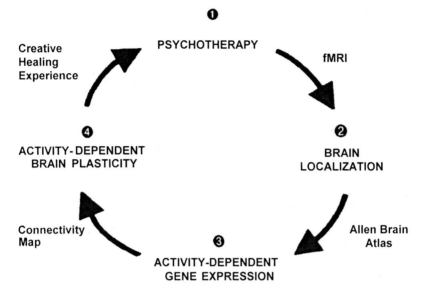

Figure 2: *An* in silico *model for mind-brain-gene psychotherapy. This* in silico *model traces the circular and recursive path of information transduction between mind, activity-dependent gene expression, and brain plasticity during psychotherapy. (1) The novel, numinous, and salient experiences of consciousness in psychotherapy evokes* activity in brain neurons *that can be (2) localized in the brain with functional Magnetic Resonance Imaging (fMRI). (3) The Allen Brain Atlas then can be accessed free on the Internet to determine what profiles of activity-dependent gene expression were evoked on these brain locations by psychotherapy. (4) The Connectivity Map is another free database on the Internet that can be accessed to determine what molecular-genomic transformations within brain cells were evoked by the activity-dependent gene expression originally evoked by psychotherapy. (4) Some of these molecular-genomic transformations in brain neurons will lead to the generation of new proteins that will evoke activity-dependent brain plasticity (synaptogenesis and neurogenesis) to create new neural networks, which will stimulate and encode new and numinous transformations of consciousness, which will in turn evoke yet another recursive exponential spiral of continuing cycles of the co-creation of brain and consciousness (Rossi 1972/1985/2000, 2002, 2004, 2007).*

all the pathways between mind and gene for free with existing million dollar databases? Well, I've actually been exploring this *in silico* path for the past half a dozen years or so, and it has led to many publications (Rossi 2002, 2004, 2007; Rossi et al. 2006). But it has been tough going.

The main problem is that all the free databases that make up the *in silico* model in figure 2 were developed by biologists and neuroscientists for their own specialized world of research concerns. These biological researchers are intensely concerned with solving basic problems in medicine—cancer, organic brain diseases, immunological dysfunctions, etc. All certainly praiseworthy preoccupations. These databases are concerned with stress and its associated dysfunctions on the brain and body at the molecular-genomic level, but they are not concerned with psychotherapy. Enter terms like "psychotherapy, cognitive, creative, imaginative, and behavior" in their search boxes and they usually respond with a standard phrase indicating that they do not index these terms in their literature searches and database. In short, most of these million dollar databases of biology and medicine are still blind to psychology, psychotherapy, and the humanities.

What is now desperately needed are new psychological front ends to these *in silico biological databases.* That is, we must add to their capacity to search for the molecular-genomic foundations of our world of psychology and psychotherapy by responding appropriately to search terms such as "addiction, behavior, cognition, creativity, dance, depression, drama, genius, imagination, joy, happiness, meditation, metaphor, mythology, prayer, ritual, storytelling, spiritual, stress," etc. Certainly there is enough fundamental and applied research here for dozens of Ph.D. dissertations for expanding coverage of the biological and medical databases to include all the life sciences and humanities. We would certainly expect that our National Institutes of Health would fund such research by qualified students in the arts as well as in the sciences.

All four technologies tracing the circular, recursive flow of information transduction between mind and gene in figure 2 (i.e., fMRI, the Allen Brain Atlas, Connectivity Map) are well defined in the existing scientific literature except the first: psychotherapy. With over 500 psychotherapies cited in the current literature, it is difficult to specify which psychotherapeutic techniques we should try to localize in the brain with fMRI in figure 2. Since we are specifically looking to document psychotherapy as a flow of information transduction between mind and gene, however, the choice of psychotherapeutic techniques can be narrowed to those originally designed for this purpose. Many brief cognitive-behavioral therapies, such as *the novel approaches to activity-dependent creative work,* which I outline in chapter 10 of my book *The Psychobiology of Gene Expression* (Rossi 2002), for example, can be explored easily. These structured, permissive, and easy-to-learn psychotherapeutic techniques that now need to be documented scientifically are described as *Creative Healing Experiences*

(CHE) in the next section.

3. THE MIND-BRAIN-GENE DIALOGUES: CREATIVE REPLAY AS THE ESSENCE OF PSYCHOTHERAPY: *THE CREATIVE HEALING EXPERIENCE (CHE)*

In this section I outline a new neuroscience approach to learning and documenting what I call the *Creative Healing Experience (CHE)* (Rossi 2002, 2004a, 2007). It turns out that any novel, salient, or surprising *activity* in our social and cultural milieu impacts us by turning on what biologists call activity-dependent gene expression. Stressful *activities* and relationships, for example, can modulate activity-dependent gene expression in a manner that makes the proteins that can suppress our immune system leading to illness. This, of course, is what psychoneuroimmunology is all about. Likewise, I hypothesize, novel, numinous, positive, salient, and interesting *activities* like art, drama, meditation, music, storytelling, spiritual rituals, and psychotherapy can turn on the genes that generate the proteins that facilitate what biologists call activity-dependent gene expression and brain plasticity—the growth and transformation of the synaptic connections making up the neural networks of our brain, mind, and consciousness.

I propose that this is the psychobiological essence of what is now called Positive Psychology and what we may presume is the scientific basis of healing in Marion Woodman's BodySoul Workshops outlined in figure 1. This means that if you believe that you are initiating novel, and important *activities*, interpretations, and behavioral interventions in your client's life, then *ipso facto* you are facilitating their activity-dependent gene expression and brain plasticity!

As with any truly new theory, however, the role of activity-dependent gene expression and brain plasticity in human experience and social affairs is still controversial. *No one has yet done a single study that clearly documents how psychotherapy modulates activity-dependent gene expression and brain plasticity.* The psychosocial genomic perspectives we apply to psychotherapy here, however, are derived directly from the implications of current research in neuroscience, genomics, and bioinformatics (the sciences of biological information). Of most direct relevance for psychotherapists is the new research on how the mind, brain, and gene are constantly engaged in dialogues on unconscious (implicit) and conscious (explicit) levels (see p. 29 update).

I propose that these dialogues are an emerging model for the deep psychobiological foundation of virtually all schools of psychotherapy (Rossi 2007), which can be explored with the new complementary computer alchemy of tracing the *in silico* flow of information transduction between mind, brain, and gene, as illustrated in figure 2. Interesting and promising hypotheses initially explored and assessed very economically *in silico* can then be validated with the multimil-

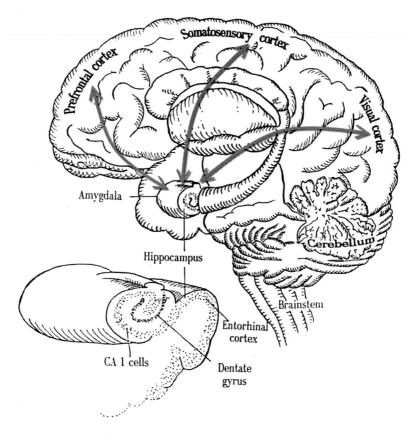

Figure 3: *The mind-brain-gene dialogues: Creative replay between the hippocampus and the cortex is the essence of psychotherapy. The enlarged cutout of the hippocampus illustrates the dentate gyrus that is a temporary storage location of new memory, learning, and behavior, which is then transferred to various areas of the cortex during the off-line creative dialogues replayed during slow-wave sleep and REM dreaming (Rossi 2002, 2004, 2007). I hypothesize that these natural off-line creative dialogues are facilitated by novel, enriching, and salient dialogues between psychotherapist and client during psychotherapy.*

lion dollar "wet-ware" biological laboratories of classical molecular medicine.

Figure 3 is a profile of the human brain with a cutout of the hippocampus, which is the part of the brain that first records a memory of anything novel, salient, or surprising. The hippocampus only makes a temporary recording of new memory, learning, or behavior, however. Later, during "off-line periods" of sleep, dreaming, and rest when the conscious mind is not actively engaged in dealing with outer realities, the hippocampus and the neocortex engage in a neural dialogue to update, replay, and consolidate the new memory in more permanent storage locations throughout the brain. *These mind-brain-gene dialogues activate and creatively replay the "local-global computations" of the cortex (Buzsáki 2007), which are now believed to be the neural correlates of consciousness long sought by the late Francis Crick* (Crick and Koch 2003).

Lisman and Morris (2001) describe how this off-line dialogue activates and replays novel and significant life experience between the cortex and hippocampus of the brain as follows:

> . . . newly acquired sensory information is funneled through the cortex to the hippocampus. Surprisingly, only the hippocampus actually learns at this time —it is said to be on-line. *Later, when the hippocampus is off-line (probably during sleep), it replays stored information, transmitting it to the cortex. The cortex is considered to be a slow learner, capable of lasting memory storage only as a result of this repeated replaying of information by the hippocampus.* In some views, the hippocampus is only a temporary memory store—once memory traces become stabilized in the cortex, memories can be accessed even if the hippocampus is removed. *There is now direct evidence that some form of hippocampal replay occurs . . . These results support the idea that the hippocampus is the fast on-line learner that "teaches" the slower cortex off-line.* (247–248, emphasis added)

I now hypothesize that this entirely natural psychobiological dialogue between our cortex and hippocampus is the essential process that we attempt to facilitate in our emerging mind-brain-gene model of creativity, imagination, and psychotherapy. From this neuroscience perspective, therapeutic suggestions, interpretations, metaphors, cognitive behavioral interventions, art, drama, music, spiritual rituals, etc. can be more aptly described as *implicit processing heuristics (highly permissive and open-ended suggestions)*, which facilitate the natural updating dialogues between our hippocampus and the cortex every day. I *propose that the conscious, explicit dialogues between therapist and client in psychotherapy are effective to the extent that they facilitate the appropriate, corresponding off-line, unconscious, and implicit dialogues between the cortex and hippocampus that daily update consciousness by turning on activity-dependent gene expression and brain plasticity.* Implicit processing heuristics in the therapist/client dialogue are explicit hints and creative cues that we use to facilitate the off-line cortex/hippocampus dialogue that evokes *activity-dependent* gene expression and brain plasticity for adaptive behavior change.

Until recently the molecular-genomic and anatomical mechanisms of activity-dependent gene expression and brain plasticity during off-line psychological states were not understood (Stickgold 2005; Walker 2006). One of the most interesting lines of research, however, has found that when mice experience novelty, environmental enrichment, and physical exercise, the *zif-268 gene* is expressed during their REM sleep (Ribeiro 2004; Ribeiro et al. 1999, 2002, 2004, 2008). *Zif-268* is an *immediate-early gene* and *behavioral-state related gene* that is associated with activity-dependent gene expression that facilitates brain plasticity. Ribeiro et al (2004) have summarized their research as follows:

> The discovery of experience-dependent brain reactivation during both slow-wave (SW) and rapid eye-movement (REM) sleep led to the notion that the consolidation of recently acquired *memory traces requires neural replay during sleep* . . . Based on our current and previous results, we propose that the two major periods of sleep play distinct and complementary roles in memory consolidation: pretranscriptional recall during SW sleep and transcriptional storage during REM sleep. . .In conclusion, *sustained neuronal reverberation during SW sleep, immediately followed by plasticity-related gene expression during REM sleep, may be sufficient to explain the beneficial role of sleep* on the consolidation of new memories. (126–135, emphasis added)

Such research documenting how *novelty, enriched environments, and exercise (mental and physical)* can initiate activity-dependent gene expression and brain plasticity is the basis of my hypothesis about *positive, creative, therapeutic replay and reconstruction during off-line periods as the essence of mind-gene healing* on a wide variety of levels, illustrated in the recursive circles of figure 4. I have noted how these three psychosocial experiences that evoke gene expression and brain plasticity are similar to the three qualities of original spiritual experience described by Rudolph Otto (1923/1950) as the *numinosum (fascination, mysteriousness, tremendousness)*. I summarize the similarity of these three psychological and spiritual experiences associated with activity-dependent gene expression and brain plasticity as the *Novelty-Numinosum-Neurogenesis Effect (NNNE)* in creative experiences and the placebo response on all levels from mind to molecule. I propose the NNNE as the creative common denominator between art and science in a new bioinformatic theory of esthetics. Experiences of art, beauty, and truth as well as Einstein's eternal mystery epistemology are the phenomenological correlates of the activation of mirror neurons, the gene expression/protein synthesis cycle, and brain plasticity via the novelty-numinosum-neurogenesis effect (Rossi 2002, 2004a, 2004b, 2007; Rossi et al. 2006, 2008a, 2008b).

From this new neuroscience perspective we can define consciousness itself as a novelty-seeking modality of psychological experience that turns on activity-dependent gene expression and brain plasticity to encode new transformations of consciousness and adaptive behavior. Experiencing the novel, numinous, and salient (the NNNE) turns on activity-dependent gene expression and activity-dependent brain plasticity, leading to an ever-expanding spiral of co-creation between the brain, mind, and consciousness that is the essence of Carl Jung's (1916/1960) ever-shifting creative connection (circumambulatio) between the conscious and the unconscious, which he called the transcendent function. This is the essential connection between the deeply humanistic world of Jungian scholarship, the classical studies of the evolution of consciousness in mythology (Campbell 1959, 1959/1968; Neumann 1962), and our current neuroscience of mind, memory, and learning via activity-dependent gene expression and brain plasticity (Kandel 1998, 2006).

More recently Richard Dawkins (1999) explores the possibility of an exponential evolutionary spiral of co-creation between mind, consciousness, and the brain, whereby *"homo sapiens'* brain size has approximately doubled every 1.5 million years" (286). He calls this the *"self-feeding of co-evolution"* (289). Dawkins speculates about the possible mechanisms of this co-evolutionary spiral between the *"software" of the mind, language, and consciousness* and the *"hardware" of the biological neural networks of the brain* but comes to no definite conclusion about them. *I propose that Dawkins' co-evolutionary mechanism between the mind and the brain is none other than the recursive feedback spiral between the novel and numinous experiences of consciousness that are capable of turning on activity-dependent gene expression and brain plasticity,* which then evokes another set of the transformations of consciousness and imagination, which in turn evoke yet another round of activity-dependent gene expression and brain plasticity, etc. (illustrated in the varying contexts of figures 1, 2, 3 and 4). To use a rather wild biblical metaphor, these figures all illustrate how "the word is made flesh" and vice versa. In mathematical language we seek to formulate a set of *recurrence equations* that express how transformations of consciousness (C) and adaptive behavior (B) are functions of activity-dependent gene expression (G.E.) and brain plasticity (B.P.) under the impact of the NNNE (http://mathworld.wolfram.com/topics/RecurrenceEquations.html).

What motivates our exploration of this co-evolutionary spiral between the software of the mind and consciousness, on the one hand, and the hardware of activity-dependent gene expression and activity-dependent brain plasticity, on the other, in psychotherapy? If people have problems it usually means they are stuck somewhere in stage two of the creative process in one area or another of their lives. This is when most people tend to fall into a crisis and come to psychotherapy looking for help. The wise therapist, however, knows that the presenting problem is usually only a ripple on the surface of the deeper waters of self-care and creative life management. Ultimately every creative individual needs to learn how to break out of previously learned limitations on all levels from mind to gene expression and brain plasticity. Facilitating this creative process is called the "breakout heuristic" in my early growth-oriented model of psychotherapy with college students, illustrated in figure 4 of the next section (Rossi 2007).

The Breakout Heuristic: Darwin's Hourly and Daily Natural Selection of Adaptive Behavior

Recent research in evolutionary anthropology is clarifying what may have been the greatest breakout saga in human history. The story begins in Africa when a small group of hunter-gatherers, perhaps just a few hundred, left their homes to migrate over the entire globe between 50,000 to 70,000 years ago. While the anthropology tells the *outer* story of the human breakout of the physical territory of Africa, psychotherapy is focused on the *inner breakout heuristic* as we all experience it on a daily and hourly basis within the living territory of our mind-brain, as the deep psychobiological basis of adaptation and behavior (Rossi 2007).

Charles Darwin, in a prescient statement on natural selection in chapter 4 of *The Origin of Species,* commented on the significance of this daily and hourly process of behavioral adaptation:

> It may be said that natural selection is daily and hourly scrutinising, throughout the world, every variation, even the slightest; rejecting that which is bad, preserving and adding up all that is good; silently and insensibly working, whenever and wherever opportunity offers, at the improvement of each organic being in relation to its organic and inorganic conditions of life. We see nothing of these slow changes in progress, until the hand of time has marked the long lapses of ages, and then so imperfect is our view into long past geological ages, that we only see that the forms of life are now different from what they formerly were *(*http://www.literature.org/authors/darwin-charles/ the-origin-of-species/chapter-04.html*)*.

We utilize current research on Darwin's natural selection of adaptive behavior to distinguish between the experience of humans and other primates at the levels of brain anatomy, neuronal activity, gene expression, and brain plasticity. This is summarized in figure 4 wherein the large outer circle presents a new context for understanding the creative process in art, science, and psychotherapy. The outer recursive cycle of figure 4 outlines the evolutionary dynamics of waking, sleep, and dreaming in the consolidation of new memory and learning as we break out of old hang-ups, perspectives, and problems (Rossi, Erickson-Klein, and Rossi 2007). The large outer circle illustrates how *(1) novel and salient experiences while awake,* ranging from trauma and stress to positive, creative breakthroughs, are (2) *replayed in a natural dialogue between the neocortex and hippocampus in the slow-wave (SW) stages of sleep,* which are followed by (3) *rapid eye movement (REM) dream sleep* wherein activity-dependent genes such as zif-268 are turned on to generate the proteins for (4) facilitating activity-dependent *brain plasticity that transforms and encodes the future orientation of constructive memory, imagination, and behavioral adaptation.*

Is it now possible to create a mind-gene biofeedback device?

A direct implication of figures 1, 2, 3, and 4 is that it may be possible to create a mind-gene biofeedback device, which I describe

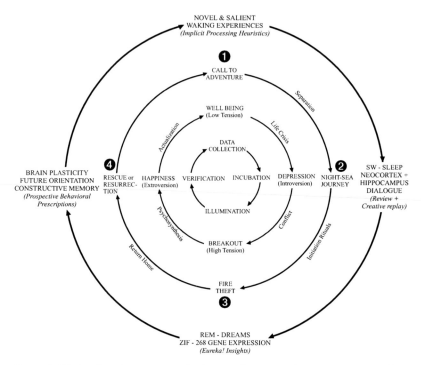

Figure 4: *The breakout heuristic in psychotherapy. The outer circle is a neuroscience update of the* four-stage creative process *(innermost circle), the* breakout heuristic during life crisis and psychotherapy *(next circle), and the* monomyth of the hero *(next circle) originally published forty years ago as a metaphor and model of humanistic psychotherapy (Rossi 2007).*

as follows (Rossi 2004a; Rossi et al. 2006):

> Will it be possible to develop a *mind-gene biofeedback device* in the future that would allow us to modulate gene expression and brain plasticity just as we now use inexpensive biofeedback devices to modulate muscle relaxation? This would be the ultimate kind of mind-body biofeedback that theoretically could facilitate to any type of psychophysiological healing at the molecular-genomic level. ... To make a mind-gene biofeedback device we need a *mind-gene transducer.* That is, we need to invent a transducer or "transformer" that converts a subjective psychological experience (thought or neural energy) into some kind of molecular signal that would turn on gene expression and brain plasticity. Recent research in nano-technology suggests how this may be possible (Rossi 2004a, pp. 304–305).

As illustrated in figure 4, we now need to assess whether we can indeed facilitate mind-gene information transduction with the breakout heuristic in psychotherapy with (1) *implicit processing heuristics* that (2) *activate* and facilitate the *natural dialogue between the neocortex and hippocampus* via the *review and creative replay* that typically takes place during sleep, dreaming, and the *novel and salient therapist/patient dialogues,* which (3) tend to *facilitate creative insights (eureka!)* that generate (4) *prospective behavioral prescriptions* that optimize brain plasticity, problem solving, and mind-body healing in psychotherapy. Let us now review the four-stage creative process in psychotherapy in greater detail before we introduce the simple and easy-to-learn approaches to Creative Healing Experiences (CHE) from mind to gene, which we now need to document with further research (Rossi 2002, 2004, 2007).

An Outline of the Four-Stage Creative Process in Psychotherapy

Stage One: Initiation—Symptom Scaling, Accessing Problems and Resources. A natural introduction to activity-dependent psychotherapy begins with the typical history-taking of the initial interview. More than mere words are involved. The typical tears and distress in an initial interview indicate that people are already accessing and replaying the important memories that signals they are embarking on a potentially healing adventure. *The therapist's main job here is to recognize that therapy has already begun and simply facilitate it.* Basic accessing questions (implicit processing heuristics) can optimize the client's inner work even before the therapist knows all the details about the problem. The therapist may begin by *symptom scaling* the patient's current emotional state. A *1 to 10 scale* (10 being the worst, 5 average, and 0 a satisfactory state) can be used to assess and validate inner work before, during, and after every psychotherapeutic encounter.

Stage Two: Incubation—The Dark Night of the Soul. Review and Creative Replay. This is the valley of shadow and doubt or the storm before the light that is portrayed in the poetry and song of many cultures. When people become stuck in stage two they fall into conflict and become agitated or depressed. This is when they are most likely to seek psychotherapy. The emotional conflicts and symptoms that come up at this time are actually mind-body language about unresolved problems at implicit or unconscious levels that require review, creative replay, and reconstruction. *The therapist's main job is to: (1)*

offer open-ended therapeutic questions (implicit processing heuristics) designed to access the state-dependent memory-encoding symptoms and (2) support the signs of arousal that are typical of creativity and problem solving. Less is often more at this stage of emotional catharsis, offering respectful listening rather than giving advice.

Stage Three: Illumination—the "Aha" Eureka Experience of the Breakout Heuristic. This stage is characteristic of the famous aha or eureka experience celebrated in ancient and modern literature when the creative process is described in the arts and sciences. Some people smile and seem surprised when they receive an unexpected and creative thought. Many patients habitually dismiss their own originality as worthless since it has never been supported in their early life. *The therapist's main job at this stage is to help the person recognize and appreciate the value of the new that seems to emerge spontaneously and unheralded.* Often the patient will have already thought of the possibilities and options that come up for problem solving at this stage but dismissed them rather than testing them in reality. Stage three is the essence of the creative process wherein I hypothesize that activity-dependent gene expression and brain plasticity are becoming manifest as the so-called aha or eureka experience of insight.

Stage Four: Verification—Reality-Testing and Self-Prescribed Behavior Change. What changes does the client want to experience as a result of this therapy? *The therapist's job here is to: (1) facilitate a follow-up discussion to validate the value of the psychotherapeutic process, (2) reframe symptoms into signals and psychological problems into inner resources,* and (3) help the client formulate a behavioral prescription for new creative cognitions and behavior. The symptom scaling of the subject's subjective state of being before and after psychotherapy can be a validation of therapeutic progress, problem solving, and healing.

Figure 5 illustrates the *four-stage creative process with hand mirroring* and the types of implicit processing heuristics that therapists can utilize to facilitate the entire process (chapter 9 of Rossi 2002). While this therapeutic process is highly structured as presented here, everyone experiences it differently. An understanding of the psychotherapeutic process and its significance is always co-creative art that engages healing dialogues between the patient and therapist rather than being a standardized procedure. To evaluate the efficacy of their creative experience, clients can be asked to estimate the intensity of how much the problem (or symptom) is experienced before and after this creative process, on a scale of 0% to 100%.

A Creative Activity-Dependent Approach to the Breakout Heuristic in Psychotherapy Illustrating the Four-Stage Creative Process

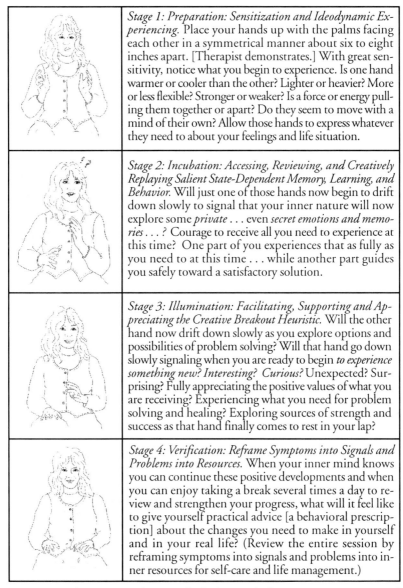

	Stage 1: Preparation: Sensitization and Ideodynamic Experiencing. Place your hands up with the palms facing each other in a symmetrical manner about six to eight inches apart. [Therapist demonstrates.] With great sensitivity, notice what you begin to experience. Is one hand warmer or cooler than the other? Lighter or heavier? More or less flexible? Stronger or weaker? Is a force or energy pulling them together or apart? Do they seem to move with a mind of their own? Allow those hands to express whatever they need to about your feelings and life situation.
	Stage 2: Incubation: Accessing, Reviewing, and Creatively Replaying Salient State-Dependent Memory, Learning, and Behavior. Will just one of those hands now begin to drift down slowly to signal that your inner nature will now explore some *private . . .* even *secret emotions and memories . . . ?* Courage to receive all you need to experience at this time? One part of you experiences that as fully as you need to at this time . . . while another part guides you safely toward a satisfactory solution.
	Stage 3: Illumination: Facilitating, Supporting and Appreciating the Creative Breakout Heuristic. Will the other hand now drift down slowly as you explore options and possibilities of problem solving? Will that hand go down slowly signaling when you are ready to begin *to experience something new? Interesting? Curious?* Unexpected? Surprising? Fully appreciating the positive values of what you are receiving? Experiencing what you need for problem solving and healing? Exploring sources of strength and success as that hand finally comes to rest in your lap?
	Stage 4: Verification: Reframe Symptoms into Signals and Problems into Resources. When your inner mind knows you can continue these positive developments and when you can enjoy taking a break several times a day to review and strengthen your progress, what will it feel like to give yourself practical advice [a behavioral prescription] about the changes you need to make in yourself and in your real life? (Review the entire session by reframing symptoms into signals and problems into inner resources for self-care and life management.)

Figure 5: *Implicit processing heuristics for facilitating the four-stage creative process with hand mirroring. This illustrates one of ten easy-to-learn novel and alternative approaches to creative psychotherapy (Rossi 2002, chapter 10).*

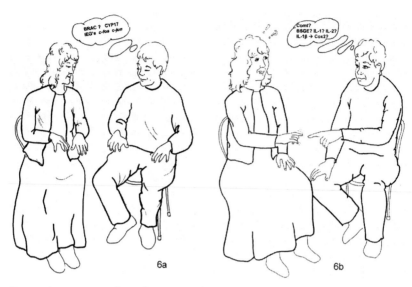

Figure 6: *An activity-dependent approach to the breakout heuristic in psychotherapy. This illustrates an emerging model of the mind-gene approach to psychodynamic psychotherapy (Rossi 2002, 2004, 2007).*

Figure 6 illustrates a highly permissive, psychodynamic, and un-structured approach to psychotherapy originally derived from Ericksonian therapeutic hypnosis. This approach utilizes the client's own spontaneous ongoing behavior rather than the more highly struc-tured approach illustrated in figure 5 (see Rossi 2002, chapter 10, for more novel, alternative approaches). It requires more extensive professional training to recognize and utilize the client's minimal mind-body language as symbolic cues and calls for the implicit pro-cessing heuristics that are now needed to facilitate the mind-brain dialogues of problem solving and healing.

The therapist's mirror neuron system needs to be empathetically alert to facilitate the constantly shifting borderline between the four stages of the creative experience (Rossi 2007). In everyday life people rarely progress through the four stages of the creative process in the idealized order illustrated in figures 4 and 5. Clients typically shift spontaneously between stages two and three with varying degrees of creative uncertainty, confusion, discomfort, and/or excitement. Some-times psychosomatic symptoms are momentarily experienced more vividly. Such transitional states of the breakout heuristic can even be

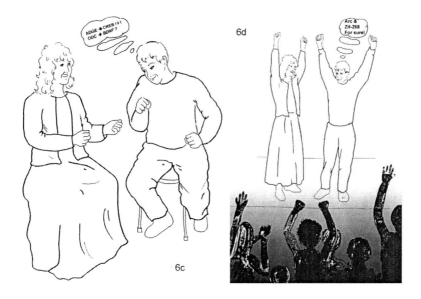

experienced as mini-emotional crises. This is well-illustrated in chapters 7 and 8 of *The Psychobiology of Gene Expression* (Rossi 2002), which provides a verbatim transcript and psychodynamic analysis of a one-hour videotape from which figure 6 is drawn. "A sensitive fail-safe approach to therapeutic hypnosis" (IC-92-D-V8) is available to students and professionals from the Milton H. Erickson Foundation (Office@erickson-foundation.org; www.erickson-foundation.org.)

Figure 6 is an artistic sketch of how a volunteer client with rheumatoid arthritis experienced the four-stage creative process of psychotherapy in front of a large professional audience of her peers. The thought balloons of the therapist are his conjectures of what the client may be experiencing on all levels, from the molecular-genomic to the cognitive-emotional-behavioral. Research is now required to assess these conjectures with the construction of standardized profiles of the four-stage creative process validated with fMRI, DNA microarrays, the Connectivity Map, etc. (Rossi 1972/2000, 2004a, 2007). Note that we are calling for measurements of the *ongoing creative process of psychotherapy*—not the measurement of *fixed traits* so typical of existing psychological scales and tests.

The Psychosocial and Cultural Genomics of Activity-Dependent Gene Expression and Brain Plasticity

The final image in figure 6 was drawn from a live *action* scene of an enthusiastic response by an audience of thousands of professionals who witnessed this videotaped demonstration at an Ericksonian congress of psychotherapy. Such a positive enthusiastic response requires some comment. Why do we have audiences to witness therapeutic process or, more generally, to participate in significant artistic and dramatic social events ranging from secular business and political meetings to the spiritual rituals of most cultures? It is generally believed that such audiences are there for education, to support a cause, etc. But what could actually be happening at a deep psychobiological level?

I offer figure 7 as a highly speculative interpretation that is consistent with the psychosocial genomic perspective we are presenting. Figure 7 is the result of recent bioinformatic research on fruit flies that illustrates how activity-dependent gene expression and brain plasticity within an individual fruit fly is related to the size of the social group it is participating in. *Nothing, it seems, turns on gene expression and brain plasticity as much as the presence of others of the same species!* Of course, this is documented here for fruit flies only. Genomic researchers consider this an example of *the deeply conserved and constitutive nature of molecular-genomic experience at this psychobiological level..* This means that it is highly likely that it is a life process that is common to most species—including humans.

This generalization to the human level certainly has many interesting implications for understanding the psychosocial and cultural genomics of human behavior and society, ranging from the dynamics of personal relationships to families, group processes, the madness of crowds, politics, war, and peace. It can also provide us with fascinating insights into the seemingly uncanny efficacy of public demonstrations of brief psychotherapy that were a frequent source of amazement, discussed by the author with teaching therapists of the previous generation as widely diverse as Carl Rogers, Milton H. Erickson, and Fritz Pearls.

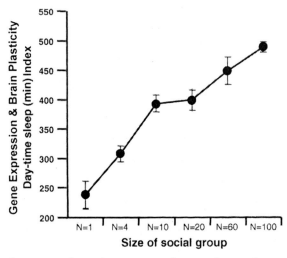

Figure 7: *Preliminary evidence of an association between the size of a social group and gene expression and brain plasticity that needs to be confirmed for humans (modified from Ganguly-Fitzgerald et al. 2006).*

SUMMARY: AN INVITATION TO OPEN SOURCE INTERNATIONAL RESEARCH

I have outlined a series of images from neuroscience and psycho-social genomics, which I propose as an emerging but still controversial deep psychobiological foundation for all the psychotherapies and medicine in general. Although this creative approach is consistent with a great deal of current research and generations of practical clinical experience, it has not been validated to meet the criteria of evidence-based medicine (EBT) and Cochran meta-analysis at this time. We therefore invite students, researchers, and clinicians to cooperate with us in evaluating these creative approaches in at least five areas that are now ripe for documentation via master's and doctoral dissertations (Rossi et al. 2006):

(1) Advance our understanding of the internal mirror neuron system and the development of consciousness via the Self-Reflectiveness Scales during dreaming and waking (Rossi 1972/1985/2000). From our new perspective, consciousness, creativity, imagination, and self-reflectiveness are the novelty-seeking *software of the mind* that facilitate a continuous, adaptive, positive, biofeedback spiral of co-evolutionary adaptation with the *hardware of the brain* via *activity-depen-*

dent gene expression and brain plasticity. This is how the mind and the brain co-create each other via the *novel and numinous activities* of art, science, drama, and dreaming in everyday life as well as in psychotherapy.

(2) Construct new psychological processing scales for measuring *the Creative Healing Experiences (CHE),* as illustrated with their many innovative and novel numinous variations (Rossi 2002, chapter 10). The Creative Healing Experiences are easily learned modules of psychotherapy that enable both client and therapist to continually assess the efficacy of their ongoing co-creative work in facilitating activity-dependent gene expression and brain plasticity for problem solving and healing.

(3) Evaluate the four-stage creative process of mind-body healing with the combined resources of CHE process and the *in silico technologies* of functional Magnetic Resonance Imaging (fMRI), the Allen Brain Atlas (ABA) of Gene Expression, and the Connectivity Map on the Internet. Utilize such research to update our understanding of medicine, psychotherapy, and rehabilitation as co-creative processes of daily adaptation whereby mind, brain, and gene are engaged in positive and constructive dialogues of self-creation at the levels of activity-dependent gene expression, brain plasticity, and adaptive behavior.

(4) In language-discrete mathematics we seek to formulate a set of *recurrence equations* indicating how *in silico* data of the transformations of consciousness (C) and adaptive behavior (B) can be expressed as functions of activity-dependent gene expression (G.E.) and brain plasticity (B.P.) under the impact of the Novelty-Numinosum-Neurogenesis Effect (NNNE).

(5) The most profound implication of research on mind-brain-gene communication, as illustrated in the recursive cycles of figures 1, 2, 3, and 4 of this chapter, is that it may now be possible to create a mind-gene biofeedback device to more precisely facilitate problem solving and mind-body healing in psychotherapy, rehabilitation, and medicine. I hypothesize that not all genes can be accessed and turned on by such a mind-gene biofeedback device but, rather, only those *activity-dependent genes* that nature is already turning on and off during our normal everyday *activities* while awake, asleep, or dreaming. The range and possible clinical applications of a mind-gene biofeedback device are completely unknown at this time. This is a challenge to be explored in experimental and *in silico* research by a new generation of students.

So much to do, so little time to explore these profound avenues of research on how the mind and brain daily and hourly co-create each other. This research is all doable right now, however, as a new neuroscience approach to unfolding the classical mysteries of consciousness, creativity, imagination, individuation, and healing in psychotherapy and medicine in the future.

Psychosocial Genomics 2009 Update

Since the original presentation of this chapter a number of outstanding papers have been published on the psychosocial genomics of dreaming (Ribeiro et al. 2008), meditation (Dusek et al. 2008), and therapeutic hypnosis (Lichtenberg et al. 2000, 2004; Rossi et al. 2008a & b). These papers all document how psychological processes can turn on gene expression and, by implication, brain plasticity (synaptogenesis and neurogenesis, Rossi 2009).

REFERENCES

Bagosklonny, M. and A. Pardee. 2002. Conceptual biology: Unearthing the gems. *Nature* 416: 373.

Buzsáki, G. 2007. The structure of consciousness. *Nature* 446: 267.

Campbell, J. 1956. *The hero with a thousand faces.* Cleveland, OH: World.

————. 1962/1968. *The masks of God.* N.Y.: Viking.

Crick, F. and C. Koch. 2003. A framework for consciousness. *Nature Neuroscience* 6 (2): 119–126.

Dawkins, R. 1999. *Unweaving the rainbow.* N.Y.: Penguin Books, 286–313.

Dusek J, Hasan H, Wohlhueter A, Bhasin M, Zerbini L, Joseph M, Benson H, Libermann T. Genomic Counter-Stress Changes Induced by the Relaxation Response. (2008). *PLoS ONE,* 3(7): e2576. doi:10.1371/journal.pone. 0002576.

Fogassi, L., P. Ferrari, B. Gesierich, S. Rozzi, F. Chersi, and G. Rizzolatti. 2005. Parietal lobe: From action organization to intention understanding. *Science* 308: 662–667.

Gallese, V., L. Fadiga, L. Fogassi, and G. Rizzolatti. 1996. Action recognition in the premotor cortex. *Brain* 119: 593–609.

Ganguly-Fitzgerald, I., J. Donlea, P. Shaw. 2006. Waking experience affects sleep need in *Drosophila. Science* 313: 1775–1781.

Iacoboni, M., I. Molnar-Szakacs, V. Gallese, G. Buccino, J. Mazziotta, and G. Rizzolatti. 2005. Grasping the intentions of others with one's own mirror neuron system. *PLoS Biology* 3 (3): 529–535.

Jung, C. 1916/1960. The transcendent function. *The structure and dynamics of the psyche,* trans. R. F. C. Hull, vol. 8 of *The collected works of C. G. Jung.* Princeton, NJ: Princeton Univ. Press, 67–91, hereafter abbreviated as *CW* followed by volume number and page number.

———. 1918/1966. The synthetic or constructive method. *Two Essays on Analytical Psychology, CW 7,* 80–89.

Kandel, E. 1998. A new intellectual framework for psychiatry? *American J. Psychiatry,* 155: 457–469.

Kandel, E. 2006. *In search of memory.* NY: W.W. Norton.

Lamb, J., E. Crawford, D. Peck, J. Modell, I. Blat, M. Wrobel, J. Lerner, J. Brunet, A. Subramanian, K. Ross, M. Reich, H. Hieronymus, G. Wei, S. Armstrong, S. Haggarty, P. Clemons, R. Wei, S. Carr, E. Lander, and T. Golub. 2006. The connectivity map: Using gene-expression signatures to connect small molecules, genes, and disease. Science 313: 1929–1935.

Lichtenberg P, Bachner-Melman R, Gritsenko I, Ebstein R. 2000. Exploratory association study between catechol-O-methyltransferase (COMT) high/low enzyme activity polymorphism and hypnotizability. *American J. Medical Genetics,* 96:771-774.

Lichtenberg P, Bachner-Melman R, Ebstein R, Crawford H. Hypnotic susceptibility: multidimensional relationships with Cloninger's Tridimensional Personality Questionnaire, COMT polymorphisms, absorption, and attentional characteristics. (2004). *International Journal Clinical of Experimental Hypnosis,* 52:47-72.

Lisman, J. and G. Morris. 2001. Why is the cortex a slow learner? *Nature* 410: 248–249.

Liu, C. , Y. Kim, J. Ren, F. Eichler, B. Rosen, and P. Liu. 2007. Imaging cerebral gene transcripts in live animals. *Journal of Neuroscience* 27: 713–722.

Lloyd, D. and E. Rossi, eds. 1992. *Ultradian rhythms in life processes: An inquiry into fundamental principles of chronobiology and psychobiology.* New York: Springer-Verlag.

Lloyd, D. and E. Rossi, eds. 2008. *Ultradian rhythms from molecules to mind: A new vision of life.* New York: Springer.

Miller, G. 2005. Reflecting on another's mind. *Science* 308: 945–947.

Moffitt, A. 1994. The creation of self in dreaming, *Psychological Perspectives* 30: 42–69.

Moffitt, A., R. Hoffmann, R. Wells, R. Armitage, R. Pigeau, and J. Shearer. 1982. Individual differences among pre and post-awakening EEG correlates of dream reports from different stages of sleep. *The Psychiatric Journal of the University of Ottawa* 7: 111–125.

Moffit, A., R. Hoffmann, J. Mullington, S. Purcell, R. Pigeau, and R. Wells. 1988. Dream psychology: Operating in the dark. In J. Gackenbach and S. LaBerge, eds., *Conscious mind, sleeping brain.* New York: Plenum Press.

Neumann, E. 1962. *The origins and history of consciousness.* 2 vols. N.Y.: Harper Torchbook.

Otto, R. 1923/1950. *The idea of the holy.* NY: Oxford University Press.

Purcell, S. 1987. *The education of attention to dreaming in high and low frequency dream recallers: The effects on dream self-reflectiveness lucidity and control.* PhD diss., Carlton Univ.

Purcell, S., A. Moffitt, and R. Hoffmann. 1993. Waking, dreaming, and self-regulation. In A. Moffitt, M. Kramer and R. Hoffmann, eds., *The functions of dreaming.* Albany: State University of New York Press.

Purcell, S., J. Mullington, A. Moffit, R. Hoffmann, and R. Pigeau. 1986. Dream self-reflectiveness as a learned cognitive skill. *Sleep* 9(3: 423–434.

Purcell, S., J. Mullington, R. Pigeau, R. Hoffman, and A. Moffitt. 1984. Dream psychology: Operating in the dark. *Association for the Study of Dreams Newsletter* 1(4): 1–3.

Purcell, S., J. Mullington, R. Pigeau, R. Hoffman, and A. Moffitt. 1985. Reply to Webb in letters to the editor. *Association for the Study of Dreams Newsletter* 2(1): 10–12.

Ribeiro, S. 2004. Towards an evolutionary theory of sleep and dreams. *A Mente Humana* 3: 1–20.

Ribeiro, S., V. Goyal, C. Mello, and C. Pavlides. 1999. Brain gene expression during REM sleep depends on prior waking experience. *Learning & Memory* 6: 500–508.

Ribeiro, S., C. Mello, T. Velho, T. Gardner, E. Jarvis, and C. Pavlides. 2002. Induction of hippocampal long-term potentiation during waking leads to increased extrahippocampal zif-268 expression during ensuing rapid-eye-movement sleep. *Journal of Neuroscience* 22(24): 10914–10923.

Ribeiro, S., D. Gervasoni, E. Soares, Y. Zhou, S. Lin, J. Pantoja, M. Lavine, and M. Nicolelis. 2004. Long-lasting novelty-induced neuronal reverberation during slow-wave sleep in multiple forebrain areas. *Public Library of Science, Biology (PLoS)* 2 (1): 126–137.

Ribeiro, S., Simões, C. and Nicolelis, M. 2008. Genes, Sleep, and Dreams. In Lloyd and Rossi, eds. *Ultradian rhythms from molecule to mind: A new vision of life.* New York: Springer. 413-430.

Rizzolatti, G. and M. Arbib. 1998. Language within our grasp. *Trends in Neurosciences* 21(5):188–194.

Rossi, E. 1972/1985/2000. Dreams, consciousness and spirit: The quantum experience of self-reflection and co-creation. *Dreams and the growth of personality.* 3rd ed. New York: Zeig, Tucker, Theisen.

Rossi, E. 2002. *The psychobiology of gene expression: Neuroscience and neurogenesis in therapeutic hypnosis and the healing arts.* N.Y.: W. W. Norton Professional Books.

Rossi, E. 2004a. *A discourse with our genes: The psychosocial and cultural genomics of therapeutic hypnosis and psychotherapy.* Trans. and ed. Salvador Iannotti. New York: Zeig, Tucker, Theisen.

Rossi, E. 2004b. Art, Beauty, and Truth: The Psychosocial Genomics of Consciousness, Dreams, and Brain Growth in Psychotherapy and Mind-Body Healing. *Annals of the American Psychotherapy Association* 7: 10-17.

Rossi, E. 2007. *The breakout heuristic: The new neuroscience of mirror neurons, consciousness, and creativity in human relationships.* Phoenix: Milton H. Erickson Press.

Rossi, E. 2009. The Psychosocial Genomics of Therapeutic Hypnosis, Psychotherapy, and Rehabilitation. *American Journal of Clinical Hypnosis,* 31:2, 281-298.

Rossi, E., R. Erickson-Klein, and K. Rossi. 2007, in press. The future orientation of constructive memory: An evolutionary theory of therapeutic hypnosis and brief psychotherapy. *The American Journal of Clinical Hypnosis* 50:4, 343-350.

Rossi, E., K. Rossi, G. Yount, M. Cozzolino, and S. Iannotti. 2006. The bioinformatics of integrative medical insights: Proposals for an international psychosocial and cultural bioinformatics project. *Integrated Medicine Insights.* http://www.la-press.com/integmed.htm.

Rossi, E., Iannotti, S., Cozzolino, M., Castiglione, S., Cicatelli, A. & Rossi, K. 2008a. A pilot study of positive expectations and focused attention via a new protocol for therapeutic hypnosis assessed with DNA microarrays: The creative psychosocial genomic healing experience. *Sleep and Hypnosis: An International Journal of Sleep, Dream, and Hypnosis,* 10:2, 39-44.

Rossi, E., and Rossi, K. 2008b. Open Questions on Mind, Genes, Consciousness, and Behavior: The Circadian and Ultradian Rhythms of Art, Beauty, and Truth in Creativity. In Lloyd and Rossi, eds. *Ultradian rhythms from molecule to mind: A new vision of life.* New York: Springer. 391-412.

Siegle, G., C. Carter, and M. Thase. 2006. Use of fMRI to predict recovery from unipolar depression with cognitive behavior therapy. *American Journal of Psychiatry* 163:735–738.

Stickgold, R. 2005. Sleep-dependent memory consolidation. *Nature* 437: 1272–1278.

Wang, J., H. Rao, G. Wetmore, P. Furlan, M. Korczykowski, D. Dinges, and J. Detre. 2005. Perfusion functional MRI reveals cerebral blood flow pattern under psychological stress. *PNAS* 102: 17804–17809.

Walker, M. 2006. Sleep to remember. *American Scientist* 94: 326–333.

8

Clinical Implications of Neuroscience Research in PTSD

BESSEL A. VAN DER KOLK

The discovery that sensory input can automatically stimulate hormonal secretions and influence the activation of brain regions involved in attention and memory once again confronts psychology with the limitations of conscious control over our actions and emotions. This is particularly relevant for understanding and treating traumatized individuals. The fact that reminders of the past automatically activate certain neurobiological responses explains why trauma survivors are vulnerable to react with irrational, subcortically initiated responses that are irrelevant, and even harmful, in the present. Traumatized individuals may blow up in response to minor provocations; freeze when frustrated, or become helpless in the face of trivial challenges. Without a historical context to understand the somatic and behavioral residues from the past, their emotions appear out of place and their actions bizarre.

Our first neuroimaging study of PTSD[1] using a script-driven imagery symptom provocation paradigm demonstrated that imaging studies can help clarify the underlying neurobiological changes responsible for the problems with reliving, attention, and arousal characteristic of PTSD. Exposed to traumatic reminders, subjects had cerebral blood flow increases in the right medial orbitofrontal cortex, insula, amygdala, and anterior temporal pole, and in a relative deactivation in the left anterior prefrontal cortex, specifically in Broca's area, the expressive speech center in the brain, the area necessary to communicate what one is thinking and feeling. This, and subsequent research supporting those findings[2-4] demonstrated that when people are reminded of a personal trauma they activate brain regions that support intense emotions, while decreasing activity of brain structures involved in the inhibition of emotions and the translation of experience into communicable language. These and other findings related to neuronal activation in response to traumatic reminders have enormous potential for articulating the targets for effective intervention and treatment.

BRAIN AS AN ORGAN DEVOTED TO TAKING EFFECTIVE ACTION

Neuroscience research has provided important new insights into the processing of intense emotions. The laboratories of Antonio Damasio,[5] Joseph LeDoux,[6] Jaak Panksepp,[7] Steve Porges,[8] Rodolfo Llinas,[9] and Richie Davidson[10] have shown that living creatures more or less automatically respond to incoming sensory information with relatively stable neuronal and hormonal activation, resulting in consistent action patterns: predictable behaviors that can be elicited over and over again in response to similar input. Under ordinary conditions the executive and symbolizing capacities of the prefrontal cortex can modify these behaviors by providing the ability to observe, know, and predict by inhibiting, organizing, and modulating those automatic responses. This allows people to manage and preserve their relationships with their fellow human beings on whom they so profoundly depend for meaning, company, affirmation, protection, and connection.

At the end of the 19th century the British neurologist John Hughlings Jackson first proposed that the brain is hierarchically organized—from the "bottom up." The organism responds to incoming information by automatically activating emotional and arousal systems that stimulate action tendencies that can be modified by thought. The highest level of integration and coordination depends on prefrontal activity that allows the organism to flexibly adjust to the environment. Jackson proposed that "the higher nervous arrangements inhibit (or control) the lower, and thus, when the higher are suddenly rendered functionless, the lower rise in activity."[11] A similar trilevel model is also seen in MacLean's triune brain.[12]

What makes people unique in the animal kingdom is their flexibility: their capacity to make choices about how to respond. This flexibility is the result of the property of the human neocortex to integrate a large variety of different pieces of information, to attach meaning to both the incoming input and the physical urges (tendencies) that these evoke, and to apply logical thought to calculate the long-term effect of their actions. This allows people to continuously discover new ways of dealing with information and to modify their responses on the basis of the lessons they learn. This accounts for the fact that human behavior is much more complex than the purely instinctual and conditioned behavior seen in other species.

However, this capacity to respond in a flexible manner emerges only slowly during the course of human development and is easily disrupted. Small children have little control over their crying and clinging when they feel abandoned, nor do they have much control over showing their excitement when they are delighted. They depend on their adult caregivers to take action after they signal their distress. That caregiver needs to figure out what is going on and needs to change the conditions in order to restore the homeostasis of the child. Throughout the life cycle, the presence of familiar and trusted human beings continues to have a profound affect on the modulation of autonomic arousal (e.g., see Ref. 8). Children only develop autonomy when they start developing a prefrontal cortex. This allows them to appraise their internal states and to execute the actions necessary to restore disturbances in homeostasis. According to Jean Piaget, the goal of development is "decentration": having *your* emotions, not *being* them.

Adults remain prone to automatically engage in relative fixed action patterns—routine ways of dealing with life that are interrupted when the usual actions do not achieve the required results. Thwarting activates emotions—signals that something is wrong: feelings of frustration, discouragement, disgust, or rage, which, in turn, either propel people to change their course of action or to enlist the help of others. People (and animals) execute whatever "action tendency" is associated with any particular emotion: confrontation and inhibition with anger, physical paralysis with fear, physical collapse in response to helplessness, an inexorable impulse to move toward sources of joy, such as running toward people one loves, followed by an urge to embrace them, etc.

The rational mind, while able to *organize* feelings and impulses, does not seem to be particularly well equipped to *abolish* emotions, thoughts, and impulses. Neuroimaging studies of human beings in highly emotional states reveal that intense emotions of fear, sadness, anger, and happiness cause increased activation in subcortical brain regions and significant reductions of blood flow in various areas in the frontal lobe.[13] This provides a neurobiological understanding of the clinical observation that people usually have difficulty organizing a modulated behavioral response when they experience intense emotions.

Emotions occur not by conscious choice, but by disposition: limbic brain structures, such as the amygdala, tag incoming stimuli and determine their emotional significance. Emotional significance in turn determines the response, what action is taken. In other words, emotional valence decides the *physical* reaction of the organism.[5] Charles Darwin,[14] Ivan Pavlov,[15] and William James[16] all noted that the function of emotions is to take physical action. As Roger Sperry, Nobel Prize 1981, said: "the brain is an organ of and for movement. The brain is the organ that moves the muscles. It does many other things, but all of them are secondary to making our bodies move."[17] Sperry claimed that even perception is secondary to movement: "In so far as an organism perceives a given object, it is prepared to respond to it. ... The presence or absence of adaptive reaction potentialities, ready to discharge into motor patterns, makes the difference between perceiving and not perceiving."[17]

Nina Bull,[18] Jaak Panksepp,[7] Antonio Damasio,[5] and others have demonstrated that each particular emotional state automatically activates distinct action tendencies: a programmed sequence of actions that function to help the organism cope with environmental challenges. NYU neuroscientist Rodolfo Llinas summarizes the role of the central nervous system (CNS) in generating action as follows: in order to make its way in the world any actively moving creature must be able to predict what is to come and find a way to where it needs to go. Prediction occurs by the formation of a sensorimotor image, based on hearing, vision, or touch. This contextualizes the external world and compares it with the existing internal map. "The ... comparison of internal and external worlds [results in] appropriate action: a movement is made" (p. 38). People experience the combinations of sensations and an urge for physical activation as a physical feeling or an emotion.[9]

People who suffer from PTSD seem to lose their way in the world. Since at least 1889 it has been noted that traumatized individuals are prone to respond to reminders of the past by automatically engaging in physical actions that must have been appropriate at the time of the trauma, but that are no longer relevant.[19] In "the Traumatic Neuroses of War" Kardiner[20] described how WWI veterans riding on the New York subway were prone to duck in fear and behave as if they were back in the trenches when the train entered a tunnel. As Pierre Janet noticed: "traumatized patients are continuing the action, or rather the attempt at action, which began when the thing happened and they exhaust themselves in these everlasting recommencements."[21]

Neuropsychology and neuroimaging research demonstrate that traumatized individuals have problems with sustained attention and working memory, which causes difficulty performing with focused concentration, and hence, with being fully engaged in the present. This is most likely the result of a dysfunction of frontal–subcortical circuitry, and deficits in corticothalamic integration.[22,23]

Many traumatized children and adults, confronted with chronically overwhelming emotions, lose their capacity to use emotions as guides for effective action. They often do not recognize what they are feeling and fail to mount an appropriate response. This phenomenon is called "alexithymia,"[24] an inability to identify the meaning of physical sensations and muscle activation. Failure to recognize what is going on causes them to be out of touch with their needs, and, as a consequence, they are unable to take care of them. This inability to correctly identify sensations, emotions, and physical states often extends itself to having difficulty appreciating the emotional states and needs of those around them. Unable to gauge and modulate their own internal states they habitually collapse in the face of threat, or lash out in response to minor irritations. Futility becomes the hallmark of daily life.

Psychology and psychiatry, as disciplines, have paid scant attention to the deficient orientation and action patterns that are triggered by sensory input, and, instead, tend to narrowly focus on either neurochemistry or emotional states. They thereby may have lost sight of the forest for the trees: both neurochemistry and emotions are activated *in order to* bring about action: either to engage in physical movements to protect, engage, or defend or displaying bodily postures denoting fear, anger, or depression that invite others to change their behavior. Pharmacotherapy helps to address some of the neurochemical problems associated with PTSD, thereby helping to modulate some of the embarrassing and upsetting behaviors and emotions, but drugs seem to not really be able to *correct* whatever abnormality underlies these behaviors and emotions.

When clinicians rediscovered the profound disruptions in the experience of physical sensations and the automatic activation of fixed action patterns in traumatized children and adults they found themselves at a loss on how to address these deficits. One thing was clear: the rational, executive brain, the mind, the part that needs to be functional in order to engage in the process of psychotherapy, has very limited capacity to squelch sensations, control emotional arousal, or change fixed action patterns. The problem that Damasio articulated had to be solved: *"We use our minds not to discover facts but to hide them. One of things the screen hides most effectively is the body, our own body, by which I mean, the ins and outs of it, its interiors. Like a veil thrown over the skin to secure its modesty, the screen partially removes from the mind the inner states of the body, those that constitute the flow of life as it wanders in the journey of each day. The elusiveness of emotions and feelings is probably ... an indication of how we cover to the presentation of our bodies, how much mental imagery masks the reality of the body"* (p. 28).[5]

Given that understanding and insight are the main staples of both cognitive behavioral therapy (CBT) and psychodynamic psychotherapy, the principal therapies currently taught in professional schools, the discoveries of neuroscience have been difficult to integrate into therapeutic practice. Neither CBT protocols nor psychodynamic therapeutic techniques pay sufficient attention to the experience and interpretation of disturbed physical sensations and preprogrammed physical action patterns. Since Joseph LeDoux had shown that, at least in rats, "emotional memories are forever" and that the dorsolateral prefrontal cortex (dlPFC), which is involved with insight, understanding, and planning for the future, has virtually no connecting pathways to the brain centers that generate and elaborate emotions, the best therapy claimed to offer is to help people inhibit the automatic physical actions that emotions provoke—limited extinction, and helping people with "anger management" and quieting them down before blowing off the handle, such as by counting to 10 and taking deep breaths.[2]

The realization that insight and understanding are usually not enough to keep traumatized people from regularly feeling and acting as if they are traumatized all over again forced clinicians to explore techniques that offer the possibility of reprogramming these automatic physical responses. It was only natural that this would involve addressing awareness of internal sensations and physical action patterns. The closest mainstream protocolized therapeutic technique that involves such "mindfulness" currently is dialectical behavior therapy (DBT).[25] However, many non-Western cultures have healing traditions that activate and use physical movement and breath, such as yoga, chi qong, and tai chi, all of which claim to regulate emotional and physiological states. In contrast, in the West working with sensation and movement has been fragmented and has stayed outside the mainstream of medical and psychological teaching. Yet, working with sensation and movement has been extensively explored in such techniques as focusing, sensory awareness, Feldenkrais, Rolfing, the F.M. Alexander Technique, body–mind centering, somatic experiencing, Pesso-Boyden psychotherapy, Rubenfeld synergy, Hakomi, and many others. While each of these techniques involves very sophisticated approaches, the nature and effects of these practices are not easily articulated and, as Don Hanlon Johnson[26] notes, their meanings are not easily captured in the dominant intellectual categories. The closest integration of mainstream science and body-oriented therapies occurred when Nico Tinbergen devoted his 1973 Nobel Prize speech to the Alexander technique.

IMMOBILIZATION VERSUS TAKING ACTION

The notion that sensory triggers reinstate hormonal and motoric responses relevant to the original trauma raises important clinical issues: one of the most critical factors that renders a situation traumatic is the experience of physical helplessness—the realization that no action can be taken to stave off the inevitable. Trauma can be conceptualized as stemming from a failure of the natural physiological activation and hormonal secretions to organize an effective response to threat. Rather than producing a successful fight or flight response the organism becomes immobilized. Probably the best animal model for this phenomenon is that of "inescapable shock," in which creatures are tortured without being unable to *do anything* to affect the outcome of events.[27,28] The resulting failure to fight or escape, that is, the physical immobilization, becomes a conditioned behavioral response.

Joseph LeDoux and his colleagues have demonstrated that the lateral nucleus of the amygdala is the critical anatomical structure in the formation of conditioned fear memories. This structure, in turn, communicates with the central nucleus of the amygdala, which distributes its output to brainstem areas that control the response of the autonomic nervous system (ANS), while connections with the periaqueductal gray region control freezing or immobility, and connections with the paraventricular hypothalamus control endocrine responses of the hypothalamic-pituitary-adrenal (HPA) axis. LeDoux and his colleagues showed that animals that respond actively to the threat thereby divert the flow of information from the lateral amygdala to the motor circuits of the striatum for active coping, preventing the establishment of conditioned endocrine and behavioral responses.[29] Interestingly, decreased activation of the corpus striatum has been found in several neuroimaging studies of PTSD.[3,4]

LeDoux and his colleagues showed that, in rats, it is possible to redirect the fear conditioned pathway that is responsible for initiating autonomic and endocrine reactions and behavioral immobilization. When rats are given the option of physically escaping from the stimulus they lose their conditioning, even after a conditioned fear response is well established. This work suggests that action diverts the flow of information from the lateral nucleus of the amygdala away from the central nucleus to the basal nucleus of the amygdala, which, in turn projects on motor circuits in the ventral striatum. LeDoux and Gorman state: "By engaging these alternative pathways, passive fear responding is replaced with an active coping strategy. This diversion of information flows away from the central nucleus to the basal nucleus, and the learning that takes place, does not occur if the rat remains passive. It requires that the rat take action. It is 'learning by doing,' a process in which the success in terminating the conditioned stimulus reinforces the action taken."[30]

Most traumas occur in the context of interpersonal relationships, which involve boundary violations, loss of autonomous action, and loss of self-regulation. When people lack sources of support and sustenance, such as is common with abused children, women trapped in domestic violence, and incarcerated men, they are likely to learn to respond to abuse and threat with mechanistic compliance or resigned submission. Particularly if the brutalization has been repetitive and unrelenting, they are vulnerable to continue to become physiologically dysregulated and go into states of extreme hypo- and hyperarousal, accompanied by physical immobilization. Often, these responses become habitual, and, as a result, many victims develop chronic problems initiating effective, independent action, even in situations where, rationally, they could be expected to be able to stand up for themselves and take care of things. In our clinic and laboratory we have taken the findings from neuroscience about the rerouting of conditioned responses by taking effective action very seriously. Neuroscience research provides the theoretical underpinning of our work with action-oriented programs with traumatized adolescents and adults, involving improvisational theater,[31] "model mugging" (in which women who have been raped are taught self-defense and learn to actively fight off a simulated attack by a potential rapist), and other interventions that involve physical action.[32]

AROUSAL MODULATION AND CONTROL OF THE ANS

Describing traumatic experiences in conventional verbal therapy is likely to activate implicit memories, that is, trauma-related physical sensations and physiological hyper- or hypoarousal, which evoke emotions, such as helplessness, fear, shame, and rage. When this occurs trauma victims are prone to feeling that it is still not safe to deal with the trauma and, instead, are likely to seek a supportive relationship in which the therapist becomes a refuge from a life self-experience of anxiety and ineffectiveness. Learning to modulate one's arousal level is essential for overcoming the resulting passivity and dependency.

Damasio draws attention to the fact that: *"It makes good housekeeping sense that* [the brain] *structures governing attention and structures processing emotion should be in the vicinity of one another. Moreover, it also makes good housekeeping sense that all of these structures should be in the vicinity of those which regulate and signal body state. This is because the consequences of having emotion and attention are entirely related to the fundamental business of managing life within the organism, while, on the other hand, it is not possible to manage life and maintain homeostatic balance without data on the current state of the organism's body proper."*[5]

The role of the ANS in PTSD has been well studied: threat activates the sympathetic and parasympathetic nervous systems. Expo-

sure to extreme threat, particularly early in life, combined with a lack
of adequate caregiving responses significantly affect the long-term
capacity of the human organism to modulate the response of the sympathetic and parasympathetic nervous systems in response to subsequent stress.[8] The sympathetic nervous system (SNS) is primarily
geared to mobilization by preparing the body for action by increasing cardiac output, stimulating sweat glands, and by inhibiting the
gastrointestinal tract. Since the SNS has long been associated with
emotion, a great deal of work on the role of the SNS has been collected to identify autonomic "signatures" of specific affective states.
Overall, increased adrenergic activity is found in about two-thirds of
traumatized children and adults.[33–35]

The parasympathetic branch of the ANS not only influences HR
independently of the sympathetic branch, but makes a greater contribution to HR, including resting HR.[36–38] Vagal fibers originating
in the brainstem affect emotional and behavioral responses to stress
by inhibiting sympathetic influence to the sinoatrial node and pro-
moting rapid decreases in metabolic output that enable almost instantaneous shifts in behavioral state.[8,38,39] The parasympathetic system
consists of two branches: the ventral vagal complex (VVC) and the
dorsal vagal complex (DVC) systems. The DVC is primarily associated with digestive, taste, and hypoxic responses in mammals. The
DVC contributes to pathophysiological conditions including the formation of ulcers via excess gastric secretion and colitis. In contrast,
the VVC has the primary control of supradiaphragmatic visceral organs including the larynx, pharynx, bronchi, esophagus, and heart.[36,40]

The VVC inhibits the mobilization of the SNS, enabling rapid
engagement and disengagement in the environment.[41] Deficient vagal modulatory capacity has been well documented in traumatized
boys and in school children with internalizing problems.[42,43] Lack of
ventral vagal modulation is likely to contribute to the problems that
affect regulation and lack of responsiveness to interpersonal comfort
in traumatized individuals.

Power spectral analysis (PSA) of heart rate variability (HRV) provides the best available means of measuring the interaction of sympathetic and parasympathetic tone, that is, of brainstem regulatory in-
tegrity.[44] Low HRV has been associated with anxiety and depression,[45–48] with coronary vascular disease, and increased mortality,[49] while high
HRV is associated with positive emotions[50] and resistance to stress.[8]

PTSD involves a fundamental dysregulation of arousal modulation at the brain stem level. PTSD patients suffer from baseline autonomic hyperarousal and lower resting HRV compared to controls, suggesting that they have increased sympathetic and decreased parasympathetic tone.[51] When presented with mental challenges, such as arithmetic tasks, people with PTSD show more arousal and less vagal control over their heart rate.[52]

Abnormally high baseline HR can result from high tonic sympathetic activity, low tonic parasympathetic activity, or both.[53] While pharmacological control over sympathetic arousal in PTSD has been fairly well studied, the parasympathetic branch of the ANS has an independent and greater influence on basal HR than the sympathetic branch, and has been specifically implicated in cardiovascular risk factors, disease processes, and outcomes. In a recent study we found strong inverse relationships between heart rate and HRV in individuals with PTSD. A substantial proportion of PTSD patients did not have elevated basal HRs. In patients with elevated HR, there clearly was a parasympathetic contribution independent of the SNS, which supports the notion that poor vagal tone may play a significant role in PTSD.[54]

It seems that, in order to come to terms with the past, it may be essential to learn to regulate one's physiological arousal. Currently, little is known about how people can learn to do that, even though a number of techniques claim to be able to help people control their HRV. However, no study has been published to date to show how changing HRV affects PTSD symptomatology. Since lack of arousal modulation is such a dominant issue in traumatized individuals we decided to systematically study whether (1) there might be an effective way of increasing HRV and (2) whether increased HRV would be associated with improvement in PTSD symptomatology. Since yoga is a very common practice for self-care in our culture, and since numerous yoga websites claim that yoga can change HRV, we decided to see if we could verify that claim (we could find no studies to support the notion that yoga, in fact, changes HRV).*

In order to test the proposition that yoga can change HRV we built a custom version of the MEDAC System/3 (NeuroDyne Medi-

*The author gratefully acknowledges the research support of the Creative Care Foundation for this study, and the contributions of Stefanie Smith, Ali Kozlowski, and Bruce Mehler, and of David Emerson and the yoga teachers of the Black Lotus project.

cal Corporation, Cambridge, MA, USA) that allowed eight subjects to be monitored simultaneously for HRV. Data were sampled at 250 samples per sec and the interbeat inter-val (IBI) determined. Normalization of IBI values was carried out using the standard algorithms in the Log-a-Rhythm HRV analysis software, version 3.0 (Nian-Crae, Inc., Cambridge, MA, USA). The normal control yoga group *(N =* 11) significantly changed HRV over eight sessions of hatha yoga: paired samples *t*-tests were conducted to examine the effects of yoga on HRV. There was a mean improvement in SDNN of 12.8, (*SD* = 16.8; $t(8)$ = 2.287; $P \le 0.05$). Yoga significantly improved PTSD symptomatology, as measured by the CAPS: total pre–post yoga $t(10)$ = 4.052; $P \le 0.01$; CAPS reexperiencing pre–post yoga $t(10)$ = 0.5.164; $P \le$ 0.001 and CAPS avoidance pre–post yoga $t(10)$ = 2.620; $P \le 0.01$. Hyperarousal was nonsignificant in the *t*-tests). When measuring HRV from session to session the yoga exhibited a large number of movement artefacts during the yoga relaxation phase (Shavasana) throughout the active treatment phase, as well as significant peripheral vasoconstriction, which interfered with getting accurate readings of HRV in this group. This suggests that the PTSD group had muscular and vascular concomitants of PTSD that interfered with the measurement of HRV peripherally.

In another pilot study eight female patients between the ages of 25 and 55 years with PTSD were randomly assigned to eight sessions of group therapy based on DBT or to 75 min of simple hatha yoga exercises, and rated by rating on the following outcome measures: Davidson PTSD Scale, the PANAS, and Trauma Center Body Awareness Scale. Sample *t*-tests were conducted to examine the effects of yoga and DBT on various symptoms of PTSD. In comparison with DBT only the yoga group showed significant decreases in frequency of intrusions and severity of hyperarousal symptoms between time 1 and time 2 ($t(6)$ = 3.44; $P < 0.05$; $t(6)$ = 3.2; $P < 0.05$, respectively).There are no significant increases or decreases in these—these numbers mean that they are related pre–post, but say nothing about significant increase and decrease—the *t*-tests reveal no significant changes for PANAS or body awareness.

The subjective reports of the yoga PTSD group were intriguing; members of the group made statements, such as: "I have always hated my body and I learned how to take care of it," "Having grown up obese and self-conscious it was wonderful to be able to move gently," "I learned to be able to focus and sense where my body was," "I was able to go shopping and know what I needed," and "I learned for the first time how to focus."

MINDFULNESS AND INTEROCEPTION

One of the most robust findings of the neuroimaging studies of traumatized people is that, under stress, the higher brain areas involved in "executive functioning"—planning for the future, anticipating the consequences of one's actions, and inhibiting inappropriate responses—become less active. Specifically, neuroimaging studies of people with PTSD have found decreased activation of the medial prefrontal cortex (mPFC).[55,56] The medial prefrontal comprises anterior cingulate cortex (ACC) and medial parts of the orbitofrontal prefrontal cortices.[57,58] The anterior cingulate (ACC) specifically has consistently been implicated in PTSD. The ACC plays a role in the experiential aspects of emotion, as well as in the integration of emotion and cognition. It has extensive connections with multiple brain structures, including the hypothalamus, amygdala, and brain stem autonomic nuclei. Thus, the ACC is part of a system that orchestrates the autonomic, neuroendocrine, and behavioral expression of emotion and may play a key role in the visceral aspects of emotion.[58] The mPFC plays a role in the extinction of conditioned fear responses by exerting inhibitory influences over the limbic system, thereby regulating the generalization of fearful behavior,[59] by attenuating peripheral sympathetic and hormonal responses to stress,[57,60,61] and in the regulation of the stress hormone cortisol by suppressing the stress response mediated by the HPA axis.[63] Hence, dysfunction of the mPFC is likely to contribute to the arousal dysregulation in PTSD.[22] The fact that the mPFC can directly influence emotional arousal has enormous clinical significance, since it suggests that activation of interoceptive awareness can enhance control over emotions.

Clinical experience shows that traumatized individuals, as a rule, have great difficulty attending to their inner sensations and perceptions—when asked to focus on internal sensations they tend to feel overwhelmed, or deny having an inner sense of themselves. When they try to meditate they often report becoming overwhelmed by being confronted with residues of trauma-related perceptions, sensations, and emotions:[63] they report of feeling disgusted with themselves, helpless, panicked, or experiencing trauma-related images and physical sensations. Trauma victims tend to have a negative body image—as far as they are concerned, the less attention they pay to their bodies, and thereby, their internal sensations, the better. Yet, one cannot learn to take care of oneself without being in touch with the demands and requirements of one's physical self. In the field of trauma treatment a consensus is emerging that, in order to keep old trauma from intruding into current experience, patients need to deal with the internal residues of the past. Neurobiologically speaking: they need to activate their mPFC, insula, and anterior cingulate by learning to tolerate orienting and focusing their attention on their *internal* experience, while interweaving and conjoining cognitive, emotional, and sensorimotor elements of their traumatic experience.

Sarah Lazar and colleagues at the Massachusetts General Hospital recently completed an fMRI imaging study of 20 people engaged in meditation involving sustained mindful attention to internal and external sensory stimuli and nonjudgmental awareness of present-moment stimuli without cognitive elaboration.[64] They found that brain regions associated with attention, interoception, and sensory processing were thicker in meditation participants than matched controls, including the prefrontal cortex and right anterior insula. The largest between-group difference was in the thickness of right anterior insula. It has been proposed that by becoming increasingly more aware of sensory stimuli during formal practice, meditation practitioners gradually increase their capacity to navigate potentially stressful encounters that arise throughout the day. Lazar concludes that this Eastern philosophy of emotion is in line with Damasio's theory that connections between sensory cortices and emotion cortices play a crucial role in adaptive decision making.

Lazar's study lends support to the notion that treatment of traumatic stress may need to include becoming mindful: that is, learning to become a careful observer of the ebb and flow of internal experience, and noticing whatever thoughts, feelings, body sensations, and impulses emerge. In order to deal with the past, it is helpful for traumatized people to learn to activate their capacity for introspection and develop a deep curiosity about their *internal* experience. This is necessary in order to identify their physical sensations and to translate their emotions and sensations into communicable language—understandable, most of all, to themselves.

Traumatized individuals need to learn that it is safe to have feelings and sensations. If they learn to attend to inner experience they will become aware that bodily experience never remains static. Unlike at the moment of a trauma, when everything seems to freeze in time, physical sensations and emotions are in a constant state of flux. They need to learn to tell the difference between a sensation and an emotion (How do you know you are angry/afraid? Where do you feel that in your body? Do you notice any impulses in your body to move in some way right now?). Once they realize that their internal sensations continuously shift and change, particularly if they learn to develop a certain degree of control over their physiological states by breathing, and movement, they will viscerally discover that remembering the past does not inevitably result in overwhelming emotions.

After having been traumatized people often lose the effective use of fight or flight defenses and respond to perceived threat with immobilization. Attention to inner experience can help them to reorient themselves to the present by learning to attend to nontraumatic stimuli. This can open them up to attending to new, nontraumatic experiences and learning from them, rather than reliving the past over and over again, without modification by subsequent information. Once they learn to reorient themselves to the present they can experiment with reactivating their lost capacities to physically defend and protect themselves.

CONCLUSION

Interoceptive, body-oriented therapies can directly confront a core clinical issue in PTSD: traumatized individuals are prone to experience the present with physical sensations and emotions associated with the past. This, in turn, informs how they react to events in the present. For therapy to be effective it might be useful to focus on the patient's physical self-experience and increase their self-awareness, rather than focusing exclusively on the *meaning* that people make of their experience—their narrative of the past. If past experience is embodied in current physiological states and action tendencies and the trauma is reenacted in breath, gestures, sensory perceptions, movement, emotion, and thought, therapy may be most effective if it facilitates self-awareness and self-regulation. Once patients become aware of their sensations and action tendencies they can set about discovering new ways of orienting themselves to their surroundings and exploring novel ways of engaging with potential sources of mastery and pleasure.

Working with traumatized individuals entails several major obstacles. One is that, while human contact and attunement are cardinal elements of physiological self-regulation, interpersonal trauma often results in a fear of intimacy. The promise of closeness and attunement for many traumatized individuals automatically evokes implicit memories of hurt, betrayal, and abandonment. As a result, feeling seen and understood, which ordinarily helps people to feel a greater sense of calm and in control, may precipitate a reliving of the trauma in individuals who have been victimized in intimate relationships. This means that, as trust is established it is critical to help create a *physical* sense of control by working on the establishment of physical boundaries, exploring ways of regulating physiological arousal, in which using breath and body movement can be extremely useful, and focusing on regaining a physical sense of being able to defend and protect oneself. It is particularly useful to explore previous experiences of safety and competency and to activate memories of what it feels like to experience pleasure, enjoyment, focus, power, and effectiveness, before activating trauma-related sensations and emotions. Working with trauma is as much about remembering how one survived as it is about what is broken.

REFERENCES

[1] Rauch, S., B. A. van der Kolk, R. Fisler, *et al.* 1996. A symptom provocation study of posttraumatic stress disorder imagery in Vietnam combat veterans. *Arch. Gen. Psychiatry* 970–975.

[2] Hull, A. M. 2002. Neuroimaging findings in post-traumatic stress disorder. *Br. J. Psychiatry* 181: 102–110.

[3] Lanius, R. A., P. C. Williamson, M. Densmore, *et al.* 2001. Neural correlates of traumatic memories in posttraumatic stress disorder: a functional MRY investigation. *Am. J. Psychiatry* 158: 1920–1922.

[4] Lindauer, R. J., J. Booji, J. B. A. Habraken, *et al.* 2004. Cerebral blood flow changes during script driven imagery in police officers with posttraumatic stress disorder. *Biol. Psychiatry* 56: 853–861.

[5] Damasio, A. R. 1999. *The feeling of what happens: body and emotion in the making of consciousness.* New York: Harcourt Brace.

[6] Ledoux, J. E., L. Romanski, and A. Xagoraris. 1991. Indelibility of subcortical emotional memories. *J. Cog. Neurosci.* 1: 238–243.

[7] Panksepp, J. 1998. *Affective neuroscience—the foundations of human and animal emotions.* New York: Oxford University Press.

[8] Porges, S., J. A. Doussard-Roosevelt, A. L. Portales, *et al.* 1996. Infant regulation of the vagal brake predicts child behavior problems: a psychobiological model of social behavior. *Dev. Psychobiol.* 29: 697–712.

[9] Llinás, R. 2001. *I of the vortex: from neurons to self.* Cambridge, MA: MIT Press.

[10] Davidson, R. J., J. S. Maxwell, and A. J. Shackman. 2004. The privileged status of emotion in the brain. PNAS 101: 11915–11916.

[11] Jackson, J. H. 1958. Evolution and dissolution of the nervous system. In *Selected writings of John Hughlings.* J. J. Taylor, ed. London: Stapes Press, 45–118.

[12] Maclean, P. D. 1990. *The triune brain in evolution: role in paleocerebral functions.* NewYork: Plenum Press.

[13] Damasio, A. R., T. J. Grabowski, A. Bechara, *et al.* 2000. Subcortical and cortical brain activity during the feeling of self-generated emotions. *Nat. Neurosci.* 3: 1049–1056.

[14] Darwin, C. 1872. *The expression of emotions in man and animals.* London: John Murray.

[15] Pavlov, I. P. 1928. *Lectures on conditioned reflexes.* Trans. W. H. Gantt. New York: Liveright.

[16] James, W. 1890. *The principles of psychology*, Vol. 1. London: Dover Publishing.

[17] Sperry, R. W. 1952. Neurology and the mind-brain problem. *Am. Scientist* 40: 291–312.

[18] Bull, N. 1951. *The attitude theory of emotion. Nervous and mental disease monographs.* New York.

[19] Janet, P. 1889. *L'automatisme psychologique.* Paris: Félix Alcan.

[20] Kardiner, A. 1941. *The traumatic neuroses of war.* New York: Hoeber.

[21] Janet, P. 1919. *Les médications psychologiques*, 3 vols. Paris: Félix Alcan.

[22] Vasterling, J., K. Brailey, N. Constans, *et al.* 1998. Attention and memory dysfunction in posttraumatic stress disorder. *Neuropsychology* 12: 121–133.

[23] Clark, R. C., A. C. McFarlane, P. L. P. Morris, *et al.* 2003. Cerebral function in posttraumatic stress disorder during verbal working memory upgrading: a positron emission tomography study. *Biol. Psychiatry* 53: 474–481.

[24] Krystal, H. 1988. *Integration and self-healing.* Hillsdale, NJ: The Analytic Press.

[25] Linehan, M. M., H. E. Armstrong, A. Suarez, *et al.* 1991. Cognitive-behavioural treatment of chronically parasuicidal borderline patients. *Arch. Gen. Psychiatry* 48: 1060–1064.

[26] Hanlon-Johnson, D., and I. J. Grand, eds. 1998. *The body in psychotherapy: inquiries in somatic psychology.* Berkeley, CA: North Atlantic Books.

[27] Maier, S. F., and M. E. P. Seligman. 1976. Learned helplessness: theory and evidence. *J. Exp. Psychol. Gen.* 105: 3–46.

[28] van der Kolk, B. A., M. Greenberg, H. Boyd, *et al.* 1985. Inescapable shock, neurotransmitters, and addiction to trauma: toward a psychobiology of posttraumatic stress disorder. *Biol. Psychiatry* 20: 314–325.

[29] Amorapanth, P., J. E. LeDoux, and K. Nader. 2000. Different lateral amygdala outputs mediate reaction and actions elicited by a fear-arousing stimulus. *Nat. Neurosci.* 3: 74–49.

[30] LeDoux, J. E., and J. M. Gorman. 2001. A call to action: overcoming anxiety through active coping. *Am. J. Psychiatry* 1953–1955.

[31] Kisiel, C., M. Blaustein, J. Spinazzola, *et al.* 2005. Evaluation of a theater based youth violence prevention program for elementary school children. *J. School Viol.* 5: 19–36.

[32] Macy, R., L. Behar, R. Paulson, *et al.* 2004. Community-based, acute posttraumatic stress management: a description and evaluation of a psychosocial-intervention continuum. *Harv. Rev. Psychiatry* 12: 217–228.

[33] Pitman, R. 1989. Post-traumatic stress disorder, hormones, and memory. *Biol. Psychiatry* 26: 221–223.

[34] De Bellis, M. D., M. S. Keshavan, D. B. Clark, *et al.* 1999. Developmental traumatology part II. brain development. *Biol. Psychiatry* 45: 1271–1284.

[35] De Bellis, M., L. Lefter, P. Trickett, *et al.* 1994. Urinary catecholamine excretion in sexually-abused girls. *J. Am. Acad. Child Adolesc. Psychiatry* 33: 320–327.

[36] Porges, S. 1991. Vagal tone: an autonomic mediator of affect. In *The development of affect regulation and dysregulation.* J. Garber and K. A. Dodge, eds. New York: Cambridge University Press, 111–128.

[37] Porges, S. W., J. A. Doussard-Roosevelt, and A. K. Maiti. 1994. Vagal tone and the physiological regulation of emotion. In *Emotion regulation: behavioral and biological considerations.* N. A. Fox, ed. 59 (2-3, Serial No. 240), 167–186. Monograph of the Society for Research in Child Development.

[38] Porges, S., and J. Doussard-Roosevelt. 1997. The psychophysiology of temperament. In *The handbook of child and adolescent psychiatry.* J. D. Noshpitz, ed. New York: Wiley Press, 250–268.

[39] Porges, S., J. Doussard-Roosevelt, A. Portales, *et al.* 1994. Cardiac vagal tone: stability and relation to difficultness in infants and three-year-old children. *Dev. Psychobiol.* 27: 289–300.

[40] Porges, S. 1995. Orienting in a defensive world: mammalian modifications of our evolutionary heritage. A Polyvagal theory. *Psychophysiology* 32: 301–318.

[41] Mezzacappa, E., R. Kelsey, E. Katkin, *et al.* 2001. Vagal rebound and recovery from psychological stress. *Psychosom. Med.* 63: 650–657.

[42] Mezzacappa, E., A. Earls, and D. Kindlon. 1998. Executive and motivational control of performance task behavior, and autonomic heart-rate regulation in children: physiologic validation of two-factor solution inhibitory control. *J. Child. Psychol. Psychiatry* 39: 525–531.

[43] Seguin, J., R. Pihl, P. Harden, *et al.* 1995. Cognitive and neuropsychological characteristics of physically aggressive boys. *J. Abnorm. Psychol.* 104: 614–624.

[44] Porges, S. 1991. Vagal tone: an autonomic mediator of affect. In *The development of affect regulation and dysregulation.* Garber and Dodge, eds. New York: Cambridge University Press, 111–128.

[45] Carney, R. M., M. W. Rich, K. E. Freedland, *et al.* 1988. Major depressive disorder predicts cardiac events in patients with coronary artery disease. *Psychosom. Med.* 50: 627–633.

[46] McCraty, R., M. Atkinson, D. Tomasino, *et al.* 2001. Analysis of twenty-four hour heart rate variability in patients with panic disorder. *Biol. Psychol.* 56: 131–150.

[47] Rechlin, T. 1994. Are affective disorders associated with alterations of heart rate variability? *J. Affect. Disord.* 32: 271–275.

[48] Shibagaki, M., and T. Furuya. 1997. Baseline respiratory sinus arrhythmia and heart-rate responses during auditory stimulation of children with attention-deficit hyperactivity disorder. *Percept. Mot. Skills* 84: 967–975.

[49] Dekker, J. M., E. G. Schouten, P. Klootwijk, *et al.* 1997. Heart rate variability from aged and elderly men. *Am. J. Epidemiol.* 145: 899–908.

[50] McCraty, R., M. Atkinson, W. A. Tiller, *et al.* 1995. The effects of emotions on short-term power spectrum analysis of heart rate variability. *Am. J. Card.* 76: 1089–1093.

[51] Cohen, J., J. Perel, M. De Bellis, *et al.* 2002. Treating traumatized children: clinical implications of the psychobiology of posttraumatic stress disorder. *Trauma Viol. Abuse* 3: 91–108.

[52] Sahar, T., A. Shalev, and S. Porges. 2001. Vagal modulation of responses to mental challenge in posttraumtic stress disorder. *Biol. Psychiatry* 49: 637–643.

[53] Bernston, G. G., J. T. Bigger Jr., D. L. Eckberg, *et al.* 1997. Heart rate variability: origins, methods, and interpretive caveats. *Psychophysiology* 34: 623–648.

[54] Hopper, J. W., J. Spinazzola, W. B. Simpson, *et al.* 2005. Preliminary evidence of parasympathetic influence on basal heart rate in posttraumatic stress disorder. *J. Psychosom. Res.* In press.

[55] Markowitsch, H. J., J. Kessler, G. Weber-Luxenburger, *et al.* 2000. Neuroimaging and behavioral correlates of recovery from mnestic block syndrome and other cognitive deteriorations. *Neuropsychiatry, Neuropsychol. Behav. Neurol.* 13: 60–66.

[56] Shin, L. M., P. J. Whalen, R. K. Pitman, *et al.* 2001. An MRI study of anterior cingulated function in posttraumatic stress disorder. *Biol. Psychiatry* 50: 932–942.

[57] Devinsky, O., M. Morrell, and B. A. Vogt. 1995. Contributions of anterior cingulated to behavior. *Brain* 118: 279–306.

[58] Lanius, R., R. Bluhm, U. Lanius, *et al.* 2005. A review of neuroimaging studies of hyperarousal and dissociation in PTSD: heterogeneity of response to symptom provocation. *J. Psychiatr. Res.* In press.

[59] Morgan, M. A., L. M. Romanski, and J. E. LeDoux. 1993. Extinction of emotional learning: contribution of medial prefrontal cortex. *Neurosci. Lett.* 163: 109–113.

[60] LeDoux, J. E. 2000. Emotion circuits in the brain. *Ann. Rev. Neurol.* 23: 155–184.

[61] Milad, M. R., and G. J. L. Quirk. 2001. Neurons in medial prefrontal cortex signal memory for fear extinction. *Nature* 420: 70–74.

[62] Lane, R. D., and K. McRae. 2004. Neural substrates of conscious emotional ex-perience: a cognitive-neuroscientific perspective. In *Consciousness, emotional self-regulation and the brain.* M. Beauregard, ed. Philadelphia: John Benjamins Publishing, 87–122.

[63] Yehuda, R. 2000. Biology of posttraumatic stress disorder. *J. Clin. Psychiatry* 61: 14–21.

[64] Lazar, S. W., C. E. Kerr, R. H. Wasserman, *et al.* 2005. Meditation experience is associated with increased cortical thickness. *Neuroreport* 16: 1893–1897.

9

Imagination and Medicine: Reply to Bessel van der Kolk

R I C H A R D K R A D I N , M . D .

I would like to begin by offering my thoughts with respect to the theme of this weekend's conference, i.e., "Imagination and Medicine." I am a physician who currently practices as both a medical internist and Jungian analyst. Multidisciplinary practice has taught me a great deal concerning both the scope and limits of medical science. Generally speaking, modern society holds to the idea that medical science is the study of the objective realities of the body and disease. However, this is a misconception; as like all other productions of the mind, science is essentially myth. This does not imply that it is false, but rather that it is both symbol and metaphor.

Western medicine has developed in the tradition of the ancient Greek School of Hippocrates and relies heavily on Aristotelian notions. It is empirical and sensate, in that it takes the material world as a proper object of investigation. Modern medicine also adopts the tenets of Newtonian science, which means that it approaches the body through

---

This chapter is based on a reply to a lecture by Dr. Bessel van der Kolk which he replaced after the conference with the previous article found in this volume. In his talk, Dr. van der Kolk presented his view on several examples of PTSD. Dr. Kradin's argument stands by itself, even though van der Kolk's specific stories are not included in the present volume and will appear elsewhere. [Ed.]

a lens of linear determinism with reductionistic goals. In practice, this approach has proved powerful, and consequently medical science has led to many advances over the last few centuries.

However, we currently know that science is not a monolithic endeavor; rather, it is pluralistic. In the modern world, classical Newtonian mechanics exists side by side with quantum mechanics; and the universe includes phenomena best described by linear analysis, whereas others require non-linear approaches. Since the early 20th century, physicists have recognized the vicissitudes of the natural world and have developed the flexibility necessary in order to describe it accurately. Unfortunately, medical science has lagged behind in this regard. This poses a problem when the subject of investigation cannot be described accurately by traditional medical scientific inquiry. Specifically, I am concerned here with medicine's failure to recognize both the complexity and non-linearity of human physiology, and, in particular, that of the nervous system.

The complexity of neural activities is best described by methods of non-linear analyses. Non-linear or *deterministically chaotic* systems are exquisitely sensitive to initial conditions, so that minor variations can ultimately yield large scale differences. The application of linear analytical methods to complex systems makes it virtually impossible to reproduce results accurately. What has not received sufficient attention is the fact that this undermines many areas of medicine, including the clinical evaluation of new drugs (Kradin 2008). The fact is that much of what we currently hold to be true about medical practice is based on false assumptions.

Few scientists would disagree that mind depends on the activities of the nervous system. But as an emergent phenomenon, it cannot be reduced to the materiality of the nervous system. Descartes was only partially wrong in his idea of mind/body dichotomy—mind is not brain; the two are qualitatively different, just as water does not share properties with the constituent elements of hydrogen and oxygen. The reductionism of modern medicine is not valid for the description of emergent phenomena like the mind. Goethe recognized this in his response to Newton's treatise on Optics, where according to Goethe, knowing how light is bent by a lens tells us *nothing* about the experience of vision, although it may accurately elucidate how the visual system works. Obviously, these are not the same aims.

My point is that neuroscience, as currently configured, can teach us little concerning the phenomenology of mind. This may sound like heresy to my fellow physician-scientists, but it is my thesis that it is true. Furthermore, our current level of understanding of neurobiology is grossly incomplete, so that, as was the case for the alchemists, much of what we are currently engaged in with respect to neuroscience is to project our preconceived ideas and theories onto the workings of the nervous system. This may explain why when we examine the brain in fMRI and PET scan experiments, what we invariably discover is what was predicted. For example, if you are either thinking or talking, then the areas that govern these activities are activated; alternatively, if you are emotional, then the emotional centers of the brain are activated, etc. However, I am not a Luddite; I am not suggesting that we ignore the neurosciences; but I am arguing that we be aware of its limits. This can be difficult when you are viewing this subject from an inexperienced vantage point and as part of a society that over-values the scientific myth.

With this as background, I want to respond to Dr. van der Kolk's lecture. Good scientists are also good storytellers, and it is important that this audience recognize that what Dr. van der Kolk has told us tonight about post-traumatic stress disorder (PTSD), while poignant and compelling, is his personal synthesis and perspective on this field. Dr. van der Kolk's story is only one of several that attempt to explain the phenomenology of psychological trauma and PTSD. As I do not consider myself to be a primary expert on this topic, I plan merely to present some of the other current perspectives with respect to this controversial area.

Definitions are important, as without them, one may confuse "apples with oranges," and become overly inclusive with respect to a subject. Whereas I am admittedly not a fan of the current DSM-IV system of nosology with respect to psychiatric disorders, it does represent the current "koine of the realm" (American Psychiatric Association. Task Force on DSM-IV, 2000). In DSM-IV, psychological trauma is defined as "actual or threatened death, or serious injury, or a threat to the integrity of self and others that yields intense fear, helplessness, or horror." This definition leaves room for substantial interpersonal variability based on both subjective interpretation and idiosyncratic emotional reactions.

The disorder termed "post-traumatic stress disorder" is generally considered a maladaptive response to trauma. As a Jungian, it is difficult to conclude that psychopathology lacks transformative value. But for the purposes of this discussion, I will not dwell on the possible adaptive value of PTSD; instead I will attend only to its phenomenology. PTSD includes the re-experiencing of dysphoric affects, a blunting of affect, hypervigilance, startle responses, memory disturbances, guilt, and shame. Substantial effort has been made towards determining who may be at risk for developing PTSD. Implicated factors include pre-morbid personality, past or current mental illness, a history of physical or mental abuse, social isolation, peritraumatic dissociative events, changes in autonomic nervous system tone, and genetics (Breslau, Davis, & Andreski, 1995). It is also important to recognize that trauma does not invariably, or even frequently, lead to dissociation, and that dissociation rarely lead to PTSD.

Much of the controversy that surrounds PTSD is centered on how traumatic events are remembered (Ornstein, Ceci, & Loftus, 1998). Cognitive science has determined that memory is predominantly a reconstruction of sets of learned percepts recreated in real time. There is no place in the brain where memories are "stored," nor is there the likelihood that memories of any type will be isomorphic with the events that produced them. The legal profession is acquainted with this fact, and much of the controversy in this field, interestingly, occurs at the interface of medicine with the law.

Some memories are registered in consciousness, require processing by a deep cortical structure called the hippocampus, and can be consciously retrieved. These memories are referred to as either explicit, nominal, declarative, or episodic memories; but for our purposes, I will term them simply as "verbally accessible." Other memories are encoded outside of consciousness, do not require hippocampal registration, and cannot be retrieved via conscious will. These memories are state-dependent, i.e., they require sensory and affective cues comparable to those available during their encoding in order to be retrieved

Disorders of memory are common in PTSD but what causes them is controversial. Intrusive recollections or cognitions occur in up to 80% of patients with PTSD, nightmares in roughly one-half. However, the idea that the images recalled are accurate representations of actual trauma is doubtful. So-called "flashbacks" occur in a minority of patients with PTSD, and curiously they can be evoked by the same chemical substances that trigger panic attacks, e.g., yohimbine and sodium lactate. However, evidence that flashbacks accurately depict the inciting trauma is lacking. This is even truer of so-called "behavioral memories," in which patients are thought to re-enact forgotten aspects of their original trauma. Evidence to support this claim is on shaky ground at best. Psychophysiological reactions that re-create the affective experience associated with trauma, such as sympathetic nervous system activation, are common in PTSD, although ~1/3 of patients with PTSD fail to develop physiological reactions when listening to scripts that include the details of their inciting trauma (McNally, 2003).

Freud suggested that the development of a post-traumatic neurosis required that subjects remain conscious during the traumatic event (Mollon, 2000). However, up to 1/3 of patients deny awareness of their trauma, possibly reflecting primary registration of a situationally accessible memory. Narrative coherence is often fragmented in patients with PTSD, but its prevalence may be more a factor of the verbal aptitude of the subject. The size of the hippocampus, the brain structure that is important in verbally accessible memory formation, is reduced in PTSD. However, it is not certain whether this reflects an acquired or innate difference from the norm. The idea that elevated cortisol levels induced by stress might damage hippocampal neurons in PTSD is unlikely, since blood cortisol levels measured in PTSD in general have been normal. The argument that the initial trauma may induce a burst of cortisol that damages the hippocampus, cannot explain memory deficits with respect to the trauma, as acute hippocampal injury would be predicted to limit only new memory formation.

There are a number of studies that suggest abnormalities based on functional PET or fMRI scanning in patients with PTSD. The study quoted by Rauch et al showing decreased blood flow to the language centers of the brain (Rauch et al., 1996) has been adopted by van der Kolk and others to argue that narrative formation is impaired in PTSD. However, such neurocognitive experiments are fraught with difficulties, their results are often inconsistent, difficult to reproduce, and they often, as in the study by Rauch et al., do not include controls. For all of these reasons, the neurobiology of PTSD remain uncertain.

A cardinal psychological feature of PTSD is dissociation, defined as a disruption of the integrated activities of consciousness, memory, identity, and perception. This is a broad definition, and by it, most of us would qualify as "dissociated" at various times during the day. However, pathological dissociation is accompanied by derealization, depersonalization, and amnesia. In my experiences with traumatized subjects, I can definitely attest to the first two, but not to the latter. Indeed, most subjects who have experienced trauma recall vividly what has occurred. It has been suggested that amnesia may be a specific result of trauma at the hands of a loved one that leads either to an "adaptive" amnesia or a denial of the event.

Without getting into detail, I want specifically to note those areas of Dr. van der Kolk's presentation that are controversial. First, there is no consensus that trauma interferes with declarative memory. There is little agreement concerning the importance of state-dependent recall, and in this regard, there is little *a priori* reason to conclude that memories of trauma are invariant or isomorphic with the traumatic events (McNally, 2003). Memories are reconstructions, and there is little evidence to suggest that this is less true of situationally accessible memories than of verbally accessible ones. Furthermore, the idea that the situation in the clinical consulting room can sufficiently mimic the state of trauma required and access these memories directly is spurious.

I do have my own biases with respect to PTSD, but I will remain unaligned with respect to which story is best adopted with respect to this disorder. Persons interested in the science of PTSD would be served well by an in-depth and unbiased reading of the literature, specifically recalling that anecdotal experiences can be misleading. For example, we know that the earth orbits the sun, yet everyday experience would suggest otherwise. One should also be cognizant of the curious fact that mind/body disorders have a peculiar predilection to transform based on beliefs that prevail in society. It is unlikely that PTSD, as we encounter it today, existed prior to the 19th century, just as flamboyant modes of hysteria (Kradin, 1997) and epidemic levels of multiple personality disorder (Putnam, Guroff, Silberman, Barban, & Post, 1986) are no longer commonly encountered in practice.

In conclusion, I have the following suggestions for psychotherapists. Like Freud, I suggest that therapists do best to eschew the medical model, as it does not accurately apply to the study of the mind.

The primary role of the psychotherapist is to engage with what is imaginal. It is not the psychotherapist's role, e.g., to uncover "objective truths." History is important, but establishing it, as objective, is beyond the limits of the psychotherapeutic profession. Instead, therapists should continue to promote symbolic approaches, assist in the construction of meaning, and attempt to integrate affect with cognition, all in the service of adaptive behavior. Finally, the best therapy promotes creativity and the capacity to play, both of which are impaired by significant psychological trauma.

REFERENCES

American Psychiatric Association. Task Force on DSM-IV. (2000). *Diagnostic and Statistical Manual of Mental Disorders.*

DSM-IV (4th ed.). Washington, DC: American Psychiatric Association.

Breslau, N., C. G. Davis, and P. Andreski. (1995). Risk factors for PTSD-related traumatic events. *American Journal of Psychiatry* 152: 529–535.

Kradin, R. (1997). Psychosomatic symptom and the self: a siren's song. *Journal of Analytical Psychology* 42: 405–423.

Kradin, R. (2008). The Placebo Response and the Power of Unconscious Healing. London: Routledge.

McNally, R. (2003). *Remembering Trauma.* Cambridge: Belknap Press.

Mollon, P. (2000). *Freud and False Memory Syndrome.* New York: Totem Books.

Ornstein, P. A., S. J. Ceci, and E. F. Loftus. (1998). The science of memory and the practice of psychotherapy. *Psychology, Public Policy, and Law* 4: 996–1010.

Putnam, F. W., J. J. Guroff, E. K. Silberman, L. Barban, and R. M. Post. (1986). The clinical phenomenology of multiple personality disorder: Review of 100 recent cases. *Journal of Clinical Psychiatry* 47: 285–293.

Rauch, S., B. van der Kolk, R. Fisler, N. Alpert, S. Orr, C. Savage, *et al.* (1996). A symptom provocation study of posttraumatic stress disorder using positron emission tomography and script-driven imagery. *Archives of General Psychiatry* 53:5, 380–387.

Healing Space

10

Re-imagining the
Architecture of Healing

A N T H O N Y   L A W L O R

W*e have forgotten the power of architecture.* This thought thunders through my brain as I stand at the center of the Great Kiva in Aztec, New Mexico. Three-feet-thick adobe walls wrap the circular room. Overhead, massive tree-trunk beams weave a latticework roof. Stillness charges the space. My lungs release a sigh. Mind hums. At the midpoint of the ceiling, a shaft of light blasts through a square opening. Wheeling Sun churns stable Earth. Opposing forces unite and swirl. This structure was not designed by a clever ego. It did not arise from the same worldview that built the sterile new hospital a mile down the road. It is not a place of fear and wounding side effects. Instead, the kiva frames the mystery of being and becoming. It is an architecture of healing.

In the kiva that day, I saw how much of contemporary healthcare architecture embodies conflict and violence. Instead of increasing well-being, the barren corridors and rooms found in most hospitals inflict isolation and numbness. Rather than nurturing patients with connection and vibrant peace, these settings imprison them in containers of struggle and lifelessness. Given a choice, who would want to spend a minute in a modern hospital?

Contemporary healthcare facilities wound by reinforcing a core belief. They embody a conviction that we can separate ourselves from the processes of living. Disinfected, hardened medical facilities concretize the concept that body is divided from mind and mind is spilt from soul (if soul is acknowledged at all). These sleek designs personify a notion that the world is chaotic and dangerous. As a result, hospitals attempt to squeeze uncertainty into knowable boxes. They try to promote health by ensnaring vast forces of life and pressing them into images of control and predictability. The standard medical setting reflects our obsession with making a world that escapes the flow of change, natural aging, and inevitable death. Based on these wounding ideas, structures advertised as healing places are, in reality, an architecture of denial.

Buildings that actually care for health encourage us to enter uncertainty and find renewal by discovering interconnecting patterns. Within fragments of contemporary living, body and mind are mended through contact with threads of relationship. As the inclusive circle of the kiva indicates, healthcare architecture that fulfills its purpose embraces the apparent opposites of healing. Science and soulfulness, professionalism and personal connection, mechanical efficiency and organic process are not viewed as enemies but are received as participants in a dynamic unfolding of revitalization.

Since present medical institutions promote wounding by embodying a worldview of chaos and fragmentation, architecture that promotes healing must be shaped by patterns of sophisticated order and integrated well-being. Vital places of healthcare cannot come from piecemeal patching of already-disjointed facilities. New designs of vibrant wholeness can only result from re-imagining the relationship of body, mind, nature, and culture and connecting what we discover to settings for healing.

To re-envision the design of healthcare places from the ground up, we can look to the foundations of architecture in imagination. Creative thinking is the primal substance of walls, roofs, and laboratory sinks. Every detail of the room surrounding you is suffused with imagination. The chair you sit upon was born as a twinkle in the mind's eye of its designer. An inspiration for a comfortable place to sit gathered materials appropriate to the task, such as wood, metal, and fabric. Imagination then shaped them into the legs, seat, back, and arms of the chair. Want to span a river? Imagination grabs a lump of earth, presses it into a rectangular brick, and joins one brick to another. In concert, the lumps of clay form the graceful curve of an arched bridge stretching from one bank of the stream to the other.

Imagination draws ideas and emotions into concrete form. The pure geometry of a circle is the guiding idea for stadium domes and cabinet doorknobs. A line provides the organizing thought for kitchen counters and skyscrapers. Joy dances in the radiant kaleidoscopes of stained glass windows and cottage gardens. Look beyond the surface of things, and you see the force of imagination shimmering within the shape, color, and texture of every human creation.

Each nuance of form and light communicates a different quality of imagination. A church steeple speaks of hope. Steel gates filtering entry to an exclusive suburban community announce control. Neon facades along the Las Vegas Strip promise excitement and forbidden pleasures.

As our thoughts and emotions permeate every detail of buildings, they become symbols of identity. Before September 11, 2001, the twin towers of the World Trade Center were icons of economic strength,

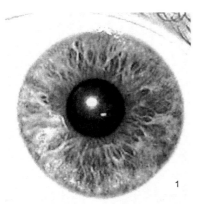

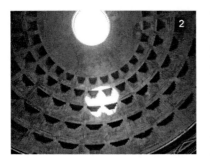

ingenuity, and aspiration. As the pair of skyscrapers burned and collapsed on 9/11, they became emblems of terror and madness. The gaping wound of Ground Zero embodied loss and sorrow.

Imagination encourages healing by linking the design of buildings to the design of our bodies. A round opening placed at the apex of a dome to receive sunlight is called an oculus. This shape mirrors the circular design of the nerves that enable the eye to perceive light. [IMAGE 1 & 2] A labyrinth's twists and turns embody the winding pathways of the brain. [IMAGE 3 & 4]

Architecture promotes renewal when it reinforces these primal connections. A hospital can

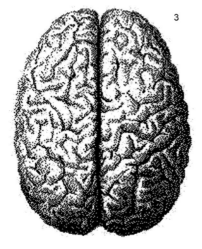

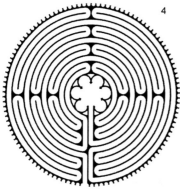

Spaciousness is the source of primal balance and healing.

serve its purpose by urging our minds to recall their symbiotic relationship with renewing processes of the body and ecology. It does so by acknowledging forces of birth, death, and renewal as they intersect the needs and dreams of our particular time and place. Imagine a maternity ward employing forms, colors, and materials that recall themes of birth, such as a rising sun, a new moon, and sprouting seeds. Take it a step further and connect these design elements to nature's births as they occur in specific locales, such as the desert Southwest, the rain forests of the Pacific Northwest, or the humid climes of Mississippi. Perhaps aging and death would seem less terrifying in settings that recognized the decay experienced each autumn as a natural current in the flow of living. By studying how various forces shape and reshape the natural world, we can discover renewing patterns of form and function. These insights can then be translated into architecture that encourages active wholeness in mind, body, nature, and culture.

Knowledge of healing forces can be uncovered by perceiving the process of imagination arising within spaciousness. [IMAGE 5] Though spaciousness cannot be seen, heard, or touched, it pervades every aspect of design and con-

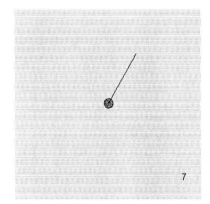

From spaciousness emerge seeds of imagination.

From seeds of imagination project rays of perception.

struction. "We build the floor, walls and roof of a house, but it is the space inside that makes it livable," explains the *Tao Te Ching*. Within spaciousness, formlessness spawns form, darkness sparks light, and silence resonates sound.

In hospitals, a passage through vitality, disease, and renewal occurs against a background of spaciousness. Screaming ambulances, beeping monitors, and churning trauma centers play out their dramas in an underlying field of silence. A recovery room's very purpose is to offer patients a spacious setting in which forces swirling through body and mind can find healing balance.

Spaciousness, appearing as form, light, and sound, spawns seeds of imagination. [IMAGE 6] From no-thing-ness emerge packets of potential thing-ness. Like a tightly concentrated seed containing the roots, trunk, branches, leaves, flowers, and fruit of an apple tree, a seed of imagination contains patterns of form and light that shape raw matter into architecture. The seed of an apple also holds the tree's shade, the rustling of its leaves, the fragrance of its blossoms, and the sweetness of its fruit. Seeds of imagination hold a design of light, sound, and form that brings architecture to life.

From seeds of imagination, rays of perception project into spaciousness. [IMAGE 7] Eyes search for light. Ears seek sound. Fingers reach toward form. As rays of perception extend into spaciousness, seeds of imagination discover varied characteristics of energy and matter. Looking more closely at white light reveals frequencies of red, yellow, green, blue, and violet. Deeper listening to a single tone dis-

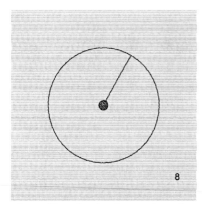

A ray of imagination draws a boundary called "world."

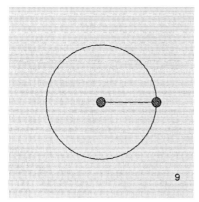

On the boundaries of the world, imagination perceives the "other."

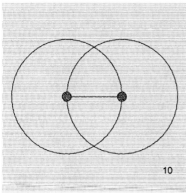

Spheres of Self and Other are defined.

closes shadings of rhythm and melody. Tracing the solids and hollows of form unearths gradations of texture.

As a ray of imagination senses the nuances of experience, it gathers light into a measurable spectrum. It coalesces sound into a harmonious scale and weaves form into beautiful patterns. This continues until the ray of imagination reaches the limits of what is seeable, hearable, and touchable. A bounding circle of perception is defined, establishing the center and circumference of the individual ray of imagination. [IMAGE 8]

Mind calls this pattern of center and circumference, this definition of known, and limits of knowing "the world." Within this structure, mind separates an individual from his surroundings. It sets one person apart from another. Imagining the world as a realm of self and other divides it into conflicting forces. Inner is perceived as opposing outer. Birth fights death. Light fends off darkness. Fullness scrambles to fill emptiness. [IMAGES 9 and 10]

This mode of perception is depicted in the image of Adam and Eve biting into the apple. The ripe fruit is torn from the tree. Its radiant skin is broken. Sweet juice spills. Shining seeds fall. The garden's harmony dis-integrates

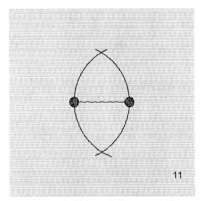

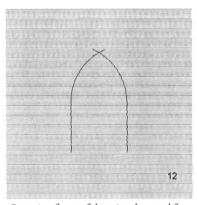

Separating Self from Other opens the primal wound.

Opposing forces of the primal wound form the portal of healing.

into a battle between good and evil, creation and destruction. Imagination distinguishes a safe self from a dangerous other. The primal wound opens. [IMAGE 11]

Peering into the gap of the primal wound, imagination perceives an abyss. The separate self conceived by the mind confronts a danger of being swallowed by an omnivorous void. To survive, self scurries to mend the wound of duality. Mind fantasizes that eliminating the other will bring a return to primal wholeness. Hypnotized by this delusion, mind seeks every way possible to control or eliminate the other. Since the other cannot exist without the self, attempting to kill the other plunges the mind into constant conflict with itself. Again and again, mind enters the fray, inflicting cycle after cycle of wounding.

Paradoxically, the primal wound of duality is also a womb of new possibilities. As the opposites of order and chaos, gain and loss encounter one another; spaciousness is churned into new forms of energy and matter.

Dueling forces of the primal wound shape the edges of architecture's first element, the portal. [IMAGE 12] The central doorway to Notre Dame Cathedral depicts this dynamic. The left side of the entry is populated with carvings of serene saints. On the right, devils dance, rattling chains and inflicting all manner of torture. At the center, sitting Buddha-like above the opposing forces, Christ raises his hand in a fear-not gesture. Instead of the nondescript entries we encounter at most healthcare facilities, patients might gain encour-

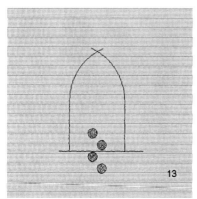

Stepping through the portal enacts the ritual of death and rebirth.

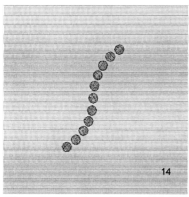

The path moves through the dual powers of wounding and healing.

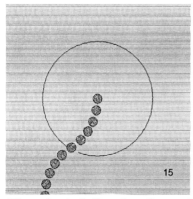

Places of arrival offer points of rest and renewal.

agement by passing through portals designed to remind them that well-being comes from the body's ability to integrate opposing forces.

Stepping through a portal's opposing forces enacts a death of the old and a birth of the new. [IMAGE 13] Like a snake shedding its old skin, architectural thresholds often display traces left by those who have already passed between conflicting powers. Doorsills worn by countless footsteps offer reassuring signs that we are not alone in our passage from one stage of experience to another. Perhaps patients entering a hospital would feel less isolated if the inward passage were marked with design forms that recall other crossings from disease to health. Recalling that a journey between opposing forces is a natural, inescapable dynamic of dwelling in the world can initiate the first stages of a healing process.

Beyond the threshold, dueling powers continue the paradoxical work of wounding and healing. [IMAGE 14] Alternating steps of struggle and breakthrough, fatigue and vitality, confusion and clarity mark the progression of body and mind through a long road of healing.

Along the way, places of arrival offer points of rest and renewal. [IMAGE 15] Fragmented and fatigued energies gather. Opposing forces rediscover their inherent unity. A new Eden is recovered. Hope for healing the primal rift between self and other glows. A new sense of center is born. As in a healing process, the conflicts experienced on the path are shed.

At each point of rest, a new seed of imagination arises. [IMAGE 16] From this new center, rays of perception spread like branches of a tree. Another bounding circle establishes a sense of center and circumference, self and other. A fresh wound of separateness opens.

This second order of wounding often shakes our faith in healing. Attempting to avoid further injury, we scramble to establish armored places of inviolable health. Attempting to distance ourselves from the varied, fluid motion of living, we build hardened, measurable structures that define direction and orientation. [IMAGES 17 and 18] Yet, structures intended to resist or imprison the processes of dissolution also block processes of renewal. They intensify the illusion of a separate self and deepen the cycle of wounding duality.

The Tibetan ritual of creating a sand mandala offers a practice for breaking the spell of this notion. During the ceremony, Buddhist monks spend up to eight days

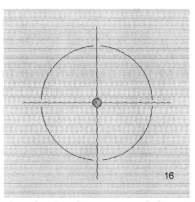

At each point of rest, a new seed of imagination arises.

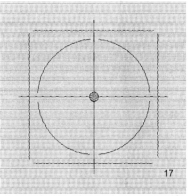

A second order of wounding causes Self to build protective walls.

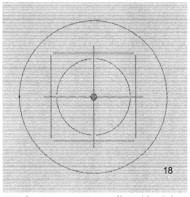

Within its protective walls, Self redefines the boundaries of its world.

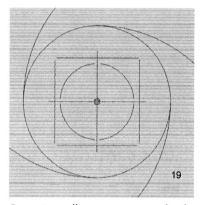

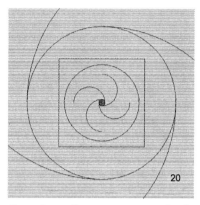

Protective wall cannot stop natural cycles of birth and death, gain and loss.

Protective walls cannot stop natural cycles of hope and fear, clarity and confusion.

sprinkling grains of colored sand to form an intricate square diagram within a bounding circle. The diagram, called a *mandala*, depicts the forces of creation dwelling in dynamic harmony. When the elaborate diagram is completed, the monks sweep the grains of the sand structure into an urn, carry the urn to a nearby river, and pour the sand into the flowing current.

Re-imagining an architecture of healing begins with seeing the flow of change as stability while seeing stability as the flow of change. [IMAGES 19 and 20] It calls for a vision of unity that embraces paradox. Your body, for example, is a unified, integrated system that maintains its wholeness through constant change. Lungs breathe, heart beats, blood flows, cells die and renew. What appears unchanging is actually constantly fluctuating. Similarly, the floor, walls, and roof of a hospital appear unmoving. Yet, throughout the day they continuously change. Sunlight sweeps a spectrum of shadows across rooms. The sounds of the day shift are different from those that resonate through the spaces at night. As you move from one room to another, view angles change.

For healthcare facilities to better serve patients, they can discover ways to embrace processes of wounding and healing. This sounds strange to the dual mind. What sane person willingly invites wounding? Yet, without daily injury to the body's existing cells, fresh cells could not bring revitalizing power.

This contradiction of creating through destroying is seen at any construction site. The earth's skin is sliced with a backhoe to open a gash that receives a concrete foundation. Trees are slashed for lumber. Stone is clawed from mountains. Iron ore and silica are boiled in raging infernos, transmuting them into steel and glass.

Instead of pretending that destruction can be avoided in the healing process, the ancient Greeks understood that seemingly opposing forces of dissolution and creation can be employed to foster dynamic well-being. They depicted this in the healing image of the rod of Aesclepius, a serpent entwining itself around a motionless staff. The snake presents a living contradiction, shedding old skin to reveal new vitality, dying to be reborn. These changes occur while clinging to an inert object. The flowing line of the serpent is interdependent with the rigid line of the rod. Psyche interacts with matter, transforming and revitalizing both.

In architecture, serpent energies entwine wood, brick, and other materials to shape vital buildings. Roofs, walls, pillars, and floors are held together by an invisible network of structural forces rising against the pull of gravity. Like acupuncture points of Chinese medicine and channels of Kundalini energy accessed by yoga and meditation, a balanced flow of energy through a building's structural system is vital to providing shelter and a sense of well-being.

Currents of energy do their revitalizing work through offering. In the sustaining cycles of nature, sunlight, water, and soil are offered to the leaves and roots of plants. Plants are offered to animals. Animals are offered to other animals. In turn, plants and animals are offered back to the soil. In this way, healing architecture provides settings for offering. In an operating room, a patient's body is offered to a surgical team. The surgeons and nurses offer their knowledge, techniques, and drugs to the patient. In the recovery room, the patient is offered to silence in which the restorative powers of the body offer healing.

A healthcare facility that invites diverse forces offers a true sanctuary of healing. It states in physical form, "We know that opposing forces cause wounding and can be frightening. Yet, this is a place that is not in conflict with conflict. It is a place that welcomes opposites to reveal hidden connections and harmony."

This healing embrace of totality has been lost in modern healthcare architecture. The traumatic journey though the healing process is tranquilized with muted colors and a rigid order of sterile spaces. At best, patient rooms are fashioned to replicate cozy bedrooms in a home. This is an admirable first step, but the mysterious, uncertain

depths of facing possible death or permanent impairment are not acknowledged. The patient is soothed, but nothing in the environment
calls to her deeper powers to face the challenge of offering her body to
the knife or to powerful drugs that can poison in order to heal.

To create healthcare facilities that face the totality of wounding
and healing, we can employ archetypal building forms. These proto-
typical design elements have been used for millennia to remind the
psyche and body that they are more than a fragmenting, isolating
disease of self against other. Such forms can help us re-imagine and
thereby restore the wholeness of mind, body, and nature that encourages genuine healing.

One combination of archetypal healing forms is a steeple and sanctuary. Steeples are not limited to churches. They rise as skyscrapers
and roof peaks. Sanctuaries are not found only in synagogues and
mosques. They receive weary souls in the privacy of a home, the quiet
bench in a city park, and the corner booth in a favorite restaurant.
The steeple offers healing power by rising from the confines of earth,
piercing the vastness of space, and offering a beacon of possibilities.
In the messy turmoil of daily concerns, a steeple calls our attention
skyward, pointing toward a freedom and peace that cannot be trapped
by the pain of illness. It points to a regenerating light that can cleanse
infections of confusion and anger. On the other hand, a sanctuary offers
healing by inviting us to reenter the womb of original wholeness, the
realm of primal unity before the duality of self and other inflicted the
first wound. Within the babel of voices crying for our attention, a sanctuary invites us to retreat and rest for a moment in its nurturing embrace. Within a sanctuary's dark shelter, the senses, mind, and body
can rest, recall their interconnectedness, and touch healing waters that
repair physical and psychological injury.

The combination of steeple and sanctuary are entered through
archetypes of portal, path, and place. As described earlier, these para-
digms of healing design support a passage from wholeness through
disease to healing.

Such design archetypes can be used as guides to imagining and
creating a healthcare facility that heals instead of wounds. To establish a place of all-encompassing healing, consider the following influences in developing a design. Connect a healing place to its particular
local and ecosystem. Study the terrain, the flow of water, the climatic

cycles of renewal, the indigenous plants and animals in order to discover forms, colors, and processes of renewal that are specific to that place. Examine how local cultural beliefs fragment or integrate a healing process; imagine how the healing place you are creating might connect these beliefs to a total view of healing. See the creation of the healing place as the birth of a living being: What does this healing place want to be? How can the individual character of this healing place be fostered to nourish and be nourished by the web of living? Use the archetypes of steeple, sanctuary, portal, path, and place to shape an environment that goes beyond being a cozy nest to powerfully acknowledge the hopes and fears of healing. How could this healing place remind patients and staff that they are not alone but are co-creators in a vital, interconnected network? Imagine ways to make the corridors of this healthcare facility reflect a process of moving from illness to health. Within the facility, provide areas for surrendering to the dissolution of the old and the revitalizing forces of the new. Face and embrace what really happens in a healing process. Re-imagine it as a poetic dance of the forces of birth, growth, decay, death, and renewal. Celebrate the beauty and mystery of the body, nature, and imagination as these engage the alchemy of birth, growth, decay, death, and renewal.

The essence of re-imagining an architecture of healing entails changing our view of walls, roofs, and other building elements. It is to let go of the viewpoint that sees them as hard, impersonal objects Instead we can see them as intimate shapes supporting shifting currents of psychological and bodily processes. To perceive hospitals and clinics as participants in healing is to shed the notion that design is a problem to be solved. It is to engage architecture as an exploration of combining multivalent forces and transcend our present grid of values and beliefs. Re-imagining healthcare facilities as places of wholeness requires that we expand the calculus of the scientific mind to include the poetry of the artistic mind. It is to take the audacious leap of experiencing emptiness, fragmentation, conflict, isolation, and other wounds of modern living as a mysterious, inexplicable process of life devouring itself to renew itself. A new healing architecture must acknowledge that its foundations rest not on solid ground but on ever-shifting currents of being and becoming. It must find innovative ways to guide seemingly opposing forces of confusion and order, unknown and known into channels of integrated healing. Ultimately, centers of genuine healing must arrange their walls and windows, doors and passages into frames of perception that point beyond themselves toward revitalizing energies ready to be born from a stillness just beyond our grasp. [IMAGE 21]

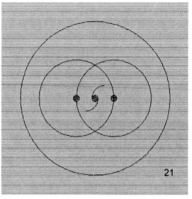

Genuine healthcare architecture embraces
healing as continuous cycles of change.

Contributor Bios

Stephen Aizenstat, Ph.D., is the founding president of Pacifica Graduate Institute, a private graduate school offering M.A. and Ph.D. programs in psychology, mythological studies, and the humanities. Dr. Aizenstat is a Clinical Psychologist, a Marriage Family Therapist, and a credentialed public schools teacher and counselor. His areas of emphasis include depth psychology, dream research, and imaginal and archetypal psychology. A major focus of Dr. Aizenstat's original research is a psychodynamic process of "tending the living image," particularly in the context of dreamwork. He extends this work in ways that engage the healing forces of dreams through imaginal "medicines." He is the author of the book *Dream Tending* (Spring Journal Books, 2009).

Lauren Y. Atlas began her doctoral work at Columbia University in September 2006. She completed her undergraduate education in 2003 at the University of Chicago, where she worked with John Cacioppo in the Social Neuroscience Laboratory. After graduating, she worked as fMRI project coordinator in Stanford's Mood and Anxiety Disorders Laboratory under the direction of Ian Gotlib, where she was involved in projects investigating the neural bases of cognitive and affective processing in major depressive disorder, social anxiety disorder, and bipolar disorder. Her graduate work with Dr. Tor Wager at Columbia takes a mechanistic approach to the study of how expectancies modulate affective experience. A central focus of her research uses fMRI, psychophysiology, and TMS to examine brain pathways mediating expectancy effects on perceived pain.

Robert Bosnak, PsyA, a Zürich-trained Jungian analyst, has since 1972 led dream groups and explored dreaming with individuals, in both analytical and didactic contexts, developing a method called Embodied Imagination: http://en.wikipedia.org/wiki/Embodied_ Imagination. Embodied Imagination, in the work with dreams and waking memories, is practiced individually and in groups in psychotherapy, medicine, theater, art, and creative research. It was a rehearsal technique of the Royal Shakespeare Company in England, and applied in medical research and psychotherapy in Japan, China, and various Western countries. Robert Bosnak has authored several books: *A Little Course in Dreams*; *Dreaming with an Aids Patient*; and *Tracks in the Wilderness of Dreaming*. His latest book (2007) is *Embodiment: Creative Imagination in Medicine, Art, and Travel*. He is past president of the International Association for the Study of Dreams and is currently based in Sydney.

Judith Harris is a Jungian analyst and yoga teacher, practicing in London, Ontario, Canada. She teaches regularly with The Marion Woodman Foundation and at The International School of Analytical Psychology in Zürich, Switzerland. She is the author of *Jung and Yoga: the Psyche-Body Connection* and of a forthcoming book, *Shattering the Vessel: The Archetype of Trauma*.

Michael Ortiz Hill is an author, registered nurse, and practitioner of traditional African medicine, a *nganga*. He has practiced as a *nganga* among Bantu people in Zimbabwe and at UCLA Medical Center. His initiation in Zimbabwe was through the diagnosis of "water spirit disease," initiation itself being ritual reconciliation with the water spirits, and has published through Elik Press two small books looking at his ordeal with multiple sclerosis as sacred illness. He is also the author of *Village of the Water Spirits*; *Dreaming the End of the World: Apocalypse as a Rite of Passage*; and the forthcoming *A Conspiracy of Kindness: The Craft of Compassion at the Bedside of the Ill*. He lives in Topanga, California with his wife, Deena Metzger, and wolf, Blue. His website is www.gatheringin.com.

Michael Kearney has over 25 years of working as a physician in end of life care. He trained and worked at St Christopher's Hospice with Dame Cicely Saunders, the founder of the modern hospice movement, and subsequently worked for many years as Medical Director of Our Lady's Hospice in Dublin. He is Medical Director of the Palliative Care Service at Santa Barbara Cottage Hospital and Associate Medical Director at Visiting Nurse and Hospice Care. He also acts as medical director to the Anam Cara Project for Compassionate Companionship in Life and Death in Bend, Oregon. Dr. Kearney is the author of *Mortally Wounded: Stories of Soul Pain, Death, and Healing*; *Spiritual Care of the Dying Patient, a Handbook of Psychiatry in Palliative Medicine*; and *A Place of Healing: Working with Suffering in Living and Dying*.

Richard Kradin, M.D., is Associate Professor at Harvard Medical School and member of the Departments of Medicine and the Center for Psychoanalytic Studies at the Massachusetts General Hospital. A Jungian analyst, he is also trained in neo-Freudian psychoanalytic psychotherapy. He is a supervising analyst and teaches courses on dream interpretation to psychotherapists and candidates in psychoanalysis. He is the author of *The Herald Dream: An Approach to the Initial Dream in Psychotherapy*, and has recently authored *The Placebo Response and the Power of Unconscious Healing* (London: Routledge, 2008).

Anthony Lawlor has practiced architecture for more than twenty-five years. He is author of *The Temple in the House: Finding the Sacred in Everyday Architecture*, and *A Home for the Soul: A Guide to Dwelling with Spirit and Imagination*. His recent film, *The Living Temple*, presents a video journey through world sacred places. Lawlor earned his Master of Architecture degree from the University of California, Berkeley. His work has been featured on OPRAH, National Public Radio, and numerous other media.

Kimberley Christine Patton is Professor of the Comparative and Historical Study of Religion at Harvard Divinity School. Her training is in ancient Greek religion and archaeology. She also teaches in the history of world religions, offering courses on comparative themes such as sacrifice, religious dream interpretation, iconography and iconoclasm, animals in myth and ritual, and weeping. She is the author of the forthcoming *Religion of the Gods: Ritual, Reflexivity, and Paradox* and *The Sea Can Wash Away All Evils: Modern Marine Pollution and the Ancient Cathartic Ocean.* She is also the co-editor of, and contributing author to, *A Magic Still Dwells: Comparative Religion in a Postmodern Age*; *Holy Tears: Weeping in the Religious Imagination*; and *A Communion of Subjects: Animals in Religion, Science, and Ethics.*

Ernest Lawrence Rossi, Ph.D., received the Lifetime Achievement Award For Outstanding Contributions to the Field of Psychotherapy by the Erickson Foundation in 1980 and the American Association of Psychotherapy in 2003. He authored 25 books and 150 scientific papers on psychotherapy, therapeutic hypnosis, rehabilitation, dreams, and the creative process. His most recent books include *The Breakout Heuristic: The New Neuroscience of Mirror Neurons*; *Consciousness and Creativity in Human Relationships*; *The Psychobiology of Gene Expression: Neuroscience and Neurogenesis in Hypnosis and the Healing Arts*; and *A Dialogue with Our Genes: The Psychosocial Genomics of Therapeutic Hypnosis and Psychotherapy.*

Esther Sternberg, M.D., received her medical and rheumatology training at McGill University, Montreal, Canada, and was on the faculty at Washington University, St. Louis, Missouri, before joining the National Institutes of Health in 1986, where she currently does research on the brain-immune connection. Dr. Sternberg is also Research Professor at American University. She is internationally recognized for her discoveries on the role of the brain's stress response in diseases such as arthritis and for her popular book on the subject, *The Balance Within: The Science Connecting Health and Emotions.*

Bessel A. van der Kolk M.D., has been active as a clinician, researcher, and teacher in the area of posttraumatic stress and related phenomena since the 1970s. He founded the first clinic in Boston, the Trauma Center, which specializes in the treatment of traumatized children and adults, in 1982. Dr. van der Kolk is past President of the International Society for Traumatic Stress Studies. He is Professor of Psychiatry at Boston University Medical School, and Clinical Director of the Trauma Center in Boston, Massachusetts. He is co-director of the National Child Traumatic Stress Network Community Program in Boston and originator of, and currently on the steering committee of, the National Child Traumatic Stress Network. Dr. van der Kolk was investigator on the first neuroimaging study of PTSD. He recently completed the first NIMH-funded study of a new exposure treatment, EMDR, for the treatment of PTSD. He was co-principal investigator of the DSM IV Field Trial for PTSD, in which he and his colleagues specifically delineated the impact of trauma across the life span, and the differential impact of interpersonal trauma. His current research is on how trauma affects memory processes; brain-imaging studies of PTSD, treatment outcome of exposure treatment vs. pharmacological interventions, and the effects of theater groups on preventing violence among chronically traumatized youth.

Tor Wager received his Ph.D. from the University of Michigan in cognitive psychology, with a focus in cognitive neuroscience, in 2003. He joined the faculty of Columbia University as an Assistant Professor of Psychology in 2004. His research focuses on the neural mechanisms involved in the cognitive regulation of emotion.

Marion Woodman, LLD, DHL, Ph.D. (Hon), is a Jungian analyst, teacher, and author of numerous books, including *Bone: Dying into Life*; *The Owl Was A Baker's Daughter*; *Addiction to Perfection*; *The Pregnant Virgin*; *The Ravaged Bridegroom*; *Leaving My Father's House*; and *Conscious Femininity*. Marion has been exploring the relationship between psyche and soma through her work and teaching for 30 years. She has developed the BodySoul Rhythms intensives to create an opportunity to study the interrelatedness of dreams and body and to share the work with the many women who are genuinely interested in this exploration. A visionary and teacher, she has developed some of Jung's ideas in an original and creative way. Marion is a founding member of the Marion Woodman Foundation, sponsor of BodySoul Rhythms Work. For more information on Marion's work, visit www.mwoodmanfoundataion.org.